Clinical guidelines for the physiotherapy management of

Whiplash Associated Disorder (WAD)

Contents

3 Physiotherapy assessment and associated issues   23

15 Further reading　　　　　　　　　　　　　　　　　　　　　　　　　100

Appendices

Tables

Figures

Evidence Summaries

Acknowledgements

The Guidelines Development Group (GDG) would like to acknowledge the following people who have contributed to the development of these guidelines:

The physiotherapists who completed the Delphi questionnaires and thus made it possible to reach consensus where there was an absence of high quality research evidence.

All those involved in the original Yorkshire project to develop a whiplash guideline in the late 1990s. Their work formed the basis for this document.

Dr. Vinette Cross, Senior Lecturer, School of Health Sciences, The University of Birmingham for section 10.

Dr Katherine Deane, Systematic Reviewer, CSP (August 2003–March 2004) for advice on Delphi methods and reviewing.

Dr. Nadine Foster, Senior Lecturer in therapies (pain management), primary care sciences research centre, Keele University for section 9.

Ralph Hammond, Professional Adviser, CSP for advice on section 7.

Dr. Sue Madden, Senior Lecturer, Oxford Brookes University for advice on Delphi methods.

Judy Mead, Head of Research and Clinical Effectiveness, CSP for supporting, managing and mentoring the CSP team throughout the guidelines development process and for contributing to the editing of the guidelines.

Andrea Peace, Library and Information Services Manager, CSP and her team for their input at all stages of the development of these guidelines.

Ceri Sedgley, Professional Adviser, CSP for her contribution to editing the guidelines.

Professor Julius Sim, Head of Physiotherapy Studies, Keele University for advice on Delphi methods including definitions of agreement.

Jackie Vokes, Professional Adviser, CSP for section 8.

The lay GDG member who used her experience of having WAD to describe her 'journey' from injury to living with WAD. Her contribution was invaluable in the production of these guidelines.

All the reviewers for their valuable comments.

Innumerable other staff at the CSP who advised and supported the team.

Executive Summary

These guidelines apply to people who have sustained a whiplash injury to their neck, aged 16 years and above. The ensuing bony and/or soft tissue injuries may lead to a variety of symptoms referred to as Whiplash Associated Disorder (WAD). Most commonly the injury will be the result of a motor vehicle collision or a sporting accident. The recommendations in these guidelines are intended to assist physiotherapists and patients in making decisions about physiotherapeutic options for interventions, following an individual's assessment.

In 2002 physiotherapists identified whiplash injury as a priority area for clinical guidelines. Following this, expert clinicians, researchers and a patient representative formed a Guidelines Development Group (GDG) to develop this document. The GDG's central focus was to understand which physiotherapy interventions are most effective in assisting people with WAD to return to normal activity. A systematic review of the literature was carried out so that recommendations for practice could be based on relevant, high quality research evidence. However, there were significant gaps in the literature. A Delphi process was therefore used to generate consensus evidence from the physiotherapy community, in order to produce more complete and useful guidelines. The GDG examined and synthesised the available evidence, interpreting its relevance for practice and developing the recommendations presented in the guidelines. The guidelines were extensively reviewed prior to their publication.

Recommendations for practice

Physiotherapists and people with WAD should be aware that serious physical injury is rare and a good prognosis is likely. Recovery is improved by early return to normal pre-accident activities, exercise and a positive attitude. Once a serious injury has been excluded, over-medicalisation is detrimental.

In the **acute stage** (0–2 weeks after injury) active exercise, education and advice on self-management and return to normal activity as soon as possible can be recommended. Manual mobilisation, soft tissue techniques, education about the origin of pain, advice about coping strategies, relaxation and transcutaneous electrical nerve stimulation (TENS) may be effective. There is no evidence to support the use of soft collars, traction, infrared light, interferential therapy, ultrasound or laser treatment.

In the **sub-acute stage** (2–12 weeks after injury) there is evidence to support a multimodal approach that includes postural training, manual techniques and psychological support. Combined manipulation and mobilisation, muscle retraining including deep neck flexor activity, acupuncture, education, advice about coping strategies, TENS, massage and soft tissue techniques may contribute to pain reduction and improvement of function.

In the **chronic stage** (more than 12 weeks after injury) exercise therapy, manipulation and mobilisation (which may be combined) and multidisciplinary psychosocial packages may be effective. Trained health professionals, who are not necessarily psychologists, can give psychological support.

Recommendations for research

During the development of these guidelines, areas for future research have been identified, based on the current gaps in existing high quality research evidence, and the clinical importance of particular research questions. These include evaluating the effect of exercise and advice given to people with WAD and treatments commonly used by physiotherapists, such as manual mobilisation, manipulation, cognitive behavioural therapy and physical agents. The relative benefits of individual or combined use of the interventions needs to be examined further. Issues relating to service delivery, prioritising patients for treatment and the natural history of WAD also require further study.

Conclusion

These guidelines are a valuable tool for physiotherapists in clinical practice, for people with WAD and for those involved in the planning, funding and carrying out of research studies. The recommendations are based on the best available evidence at the time of publication. As new evidence becomes available this will need to be considered and the recommendations reviewed. A formal update of the guidelines is planned for 2010.

Introduction

1.1 Background

In 2002 the CSP consulted its membership on priority areas for clinical guidelines development and Whiplash Associated Disorder (WAD) was one of the top 3 priorities identified.[1] Having chosen the topic the major considerations were sound guideline development methodology and working with people with WAD and specialist physiotherapists (Table 1 Appendix A). The project built on previous work carried out in Yorkshire as part of a project to develop a series of clinical guidelines (Table 2 Appendix A). In 1996 a group of over 20 physiotherapists in Yorkshire (Table 3 Appendix A) recognised the need for evidence-based guidelines for the assessment and management of people with WAD. Despite great commitment to developing the guidelines they were never endorsed by the CSP, largely because it proved impossible to carry out a full systematic review of the literature as a 'spare time' occupation. However in 2003 a group facilitated by the CSP, and including a full time systematic reviewer, set out to complete the guideline. Members of the original Yorkshire group continued to play an active part in developing this final document.

1.2 Definition of WAD

People with WAD present a variety of symptoms occurring as a result of bony or soft tissue injury caused by whiplash injury to the neck during:

- An acceleration-deceleration mechanism of energy transfer to the neck
- A rear end or side impact motor vehicle collision
- A sporting accident e.g. in diving or rugby.

    (Adapted from Spitzer 1995[2])

1.3 WAD in context

WAD is a common injury that is treated in physiotherapy clinics in the United Kingdom and beyond. It is sometimes a disabling condition and it usually occurs during transport accidents and in sporting mishaps. It is characterised by a range of signs and symptoms and can present complex challenges to clinicians. The syndrome involves trauma to a multiplicity of tissues in the cervical spine and it can affect other areas of the vertebral column. WAD can be complicated by a range of psychosocial factors. The management of people with WAD is intellectually and clinically demanding, requiring high level clinical reasoning skills. The evidence base supporting the physiotherapeutic management of WAD is in the early stages of development, but it is growing. These guidelines are designed to support both physiotherapists and people with WAD in the effective management of the condition. In addition, the guidelines highlight gaps in knowledge and indicate important questions for future research.

1.4 Epidemiology

Insurance statistics from road traffic accidents suggest that current annual incidence of WAD in the UK is approximately 300,000 new cases per annum.[3] Assuming a population of 59 million, the incidence of whiplash injuries is around 500 cases per 100,000 population per year. Incidence figures across the world are not always comparable because they are determined in different ways. However, insurance statistics suggest the incidence to be;

- 106 cases per 100,000 in Australia[4]
- 302 cases per 100,000 in Canada[5]
- 94–188 cases per 100,000 in The Netherlands.[6]

In the UK, while the numbers of insurance claims and the number of WAD cases seen in accident and emergency departments are increasing[7] the number of UK road accidents remains static.[8] It has been suggested that this discrepancy may be a result of non-organic factors such as the growing compensation culture.[9]

The UK Department of Health was approached for incidence figures but it seems that no data relating to WAD is routinely collected.

1.5 Aim and objectives of the guidelines

The aim of these guidelines is to describe a framework for the clinical practice of physiotherapy in relation to both people with acute and chronic WAD in the UK. Specific objectives were to develop guidelines that:

- Assess the quality of evidence available
- Make recommendations for future research
- Make recommendations based on the best available evidence
- Improve the quality of patient care by emphasising the best treatment options
- Are user friendly and practical
- Encourage physiotherapists to reflect on their practice
- Lead to a more consistent approach to treatment of people with WAD across the UK (although individual needs and preferences will vary)
- Are accessible for people with WAD
- Enable people with WAD to take a more active role in their treatment where they wish to do so.

1.6 Target users of the guidelines

The authors intend these guidelines to be of particular use to:

- People with WAD
- Physiotherapists of all grades working with people with WAD
- Other professionals involved in the treatment of WAD e.g. general practitioners, occupational therapists, psychologists and accident and emergency doctors
- Educational establishments, especially those with an interest in physiotherapy
- Patients and professionals living and working overseas with a personal or professional interest in WAD.

1.7 Terminology

The term 'person with WAD' has been used throughout this document on the advice of the lay GDG member. However, there are instances where the word 'patient' was more appropriate e.g. in discussing 'patient satisfaction', 'patient centred care', 'patient empowerment' or 'patient preference'.

The terms 'manipulation' and 'manual mobilisation' have been used throughout the document in accordance with the definitions that can be found in the Glossary (Appendix J).

None was declared.

GDG members are authors of papers and textbooks referred to in this guideline. This is a reflection that GDG members are experts in this field. In the first round of the Delphi process (section 2.5.3), participants were asked to list textbooks they would recommend to physiotherapists for details of assessing patients with WAD (Appendix D). This list was refined in the second round of Delphi (Appendix E) and can be found in this guideline in Section 15. GDG members did not, therefore, influence the choice of textbooks themselves.

Methods

Guidelines are a series of systematically constructed statements devised to assist practitioners with clinical decisions.[10] The process of guideline construction begins with the selection of a topic, in this case the physiotherapeutic management of WAD. The main question addressed in these guidelines is, which physiotherapy treatments are most effective for assisting people with WAD return to normal activity?

2.1.1 Scope of the guidelines

The agreed scope of this guideline was the patient journey from diagnosis to outcome, with the main emphasis on physiotherapy interventions. The scope includes people with acute and chronic WAD, physiotherapy management, issues and concerns of physiotherapists and people with WAD in the UK. It excludes children under 16 years, shaken baby syndrome.

The guidelines were developed for people with grade 0 to III WAD (section 3.2 table 3.1). However, people with grade IV WAD may present for physiotherapy assessment. For this reason signs of serious pathology (section 3.6.4) and indications for referral for x-ray, CT and MRI scan (section 3.6.5.8) are discussed in this document.

2.1.2 Role of the guidelines development group

The guidelines development group (GDG) included expert physiotherapy practitioners, a person with WAD and other relevant professionals (Appendix A Table 1). The core of the group were members of the 1999 Yorkshire GDG and experts involved in the 2001 literature search updates. They were joined by researchers and practitioners with a special interest in whiplash injury. The patient representative meant that user perspectives and priorities were high on the agenda. The group was facilitated by CSP officers, in particular, Jo Jordan, a systematic reviewer and Anne Jackson, who managed the project, designed the Delphi questionnaire and led the writing of these guidelines.

At the first formal meeting the clinical questions were defined by the GDG (section 2.2). To establish an up to date knowledge base for the GDG, a systematic review of the evidence for the most effective physiotherapy interventions for assisting people with WAD to return to normal activity (clinical question 10) was carried out. The group assessed the quality of the evidence and, where the evidence was incomplete, conducted a Delphi survey with the aim of reaching consensus. The evidence was therefore derived from:

- High quality research evidence where this was available

- Consensus opinion where the literature was incomplete or equivocal.

From the available evidence, the GDG formulated recommendations, which were tested and piloted. The completed guidelines were submitted to the CSP's Clinical Guidelines Endorsement Panel (CGEP). This publication includes a detailed description of the development process. Implementation will be an active process involving people with WAD having access to these guidelines and sharing responsibility for their care.

Figure 2.1 The guidelines development process (adapted from SIGN[11])

Select a topic

♦

Decide on the scope of the guidelines

♦

Establish a Guidelines Development Group

♦

Formulate the clinical questions

♦

Systematic review of the evidence

♦

Grade the evidence and reaching a consensus where evidence is incomplete

♦

Formulate the recommendations

♦

Test and pilot the guidelines

♦

Submission of the guidelines to the CSP CGEP

♦

Dissemination and implementation

♦

Update the guidelines

2.2 Formulating the clinical questions

At the first meeting of the GDG (18th March 2003) the clinical questions to be addressed by the guidelines were developed. These questions are listed below and the section of the guidelines where they are addressed given in brackets. Question 10 deals with the physiotherapy interventions.

1 What is the definition of WAD? (section 1.2)

2 What is the epidemiology of WAD? (section 1.4)

3 What are the risk factors associated with WAD? (section 3.4)

4 What are the mechanisms of injury of WAD? (section 3.1)

5 How can WAD be classified most appropriately? (section 3.2)

6 What are the symptoms of WAD? (section 3.5)

7 What is the prognosis and natural history for WAD? (section 3.3)

8 How should people with WAD be examined and assessed? (section 3.6)

9 What are the current guidelines in terms of pain relief for WAD sufferers? (section 3.7)

10 Which physiotherapy interventions are most effective in assisting people with WAD
    to return to normal activity?
        Acute WAD (zero to two weeks after whiplash injury) (section 4.1)
        Sub acute WAD (after two weeks and up to 12 weeks after whiplash injury) (section 4.2)
        Chronic WAD (more than 12 weeks after whiplash injury) (section 4.3)

11 Which outcome measures might be most effective for people with WAD? (section 7)

12 What are the areas surrounding litigation for physiotherapists? (section 8)

13 How can physiotherapists best educate and advise people and promote self-efficacy? (section 4.5)

14 How will the guidelines be implemented? (section 9)

15 How should we promote reflective practice amongst physiotherapists? (section 10)

16 What are the links with other guidelines? (section 11).

These questions were used to provide a framework for this document and a focus for the literature searches. Question 10 was determined to be the most important and the systematic search strategy below relates directly to this question. However a major aim was to produce a useful and practical tool for use in the physiotherapy management of people with WAD. Thus sections in these guidelines relating to clinical questions 1–9 and 11–15 contain useful background and adjunct material and put these guidelines in context. They cover the patient journey from injury, through physiotherapy assessment and onto measurement of outcome, the legal issues that may affect people with WAD, considerations of self-efficacy for people with WAD and reflective practice for physiotherapists. These sections were developed by members of the GDG, experts from outside the group and by using the results of the Delphi survey. Whilst it is recognised that these supporting sections are dealt with less systematically than is question 10, their inclusion was considered vital to producing practical and complete guidelines.

2.3 Searching for evidence

The Yorkshire Guidelines Group originally searched for literature in 1996. Further literature searches were carried out by researchers at the University of Brighton in January 2001, with updates in November 2001. Further update searches were carried out in July 2002 and February/March 2004 by the CSP's systematic reviewer.The searches carried out from 2001 started from 1995, as the Quebec Task Force[2] and other systematic reviews[6,12-15] searched for literature before this date, and these were used as the main source of studies before 1995. See Appendix B for the keywords and databases searched.

2.3.1 Outline of search strategies

The literature searches were broad. Filters to narrow the searches to randomised controlled trials or cohort studies were not used; the aim was to pick up as much background material as possible to support other sections of the guidelines. Consequently the searches were sensitive rather than specific, yielding many irrelevant citations in an effort to capture all the literature.

A final update search was carried out just before the guidelines document was completed in February/March 2004 to ensure that no studies or important documents had been published since the last literature search. A CSP librarian in collaboration with the systematic reviewer carried out this search. The search strategies that were run on Medline, Embase, AMED, CINAHL, PEDro and The Cochrane Library are shown in Appendix B. Appendix B will facilitate the searches for the update of this document in 2010.

In addition to the electronic searches, reference lists of the publications already found were examined for further relevant studies. Experts on the physiotherapy management of whiplash injuries also suggested more studies and reviews not previously found.

2.3.2 Systematic reviews

Several systematic reviews were found on the effects of treatments for WAD (Table 3, Appendix C).[2,6,12-15] After appraising the systematic reviews it was apparent that specific patient groups and interventions were not described in enough detail to enable the GDG to give the appropriate level of guidance to practising physiotherapists. Therefore the systematic reviews were used to assist in identifying the individual studies and these were then included as part of the evidence review.

Systematic reviews of the effects of interventions on mechanical neck pain, which may or may not have included people with whiplash injuries, were considered as evidence where no information was available for whiplash specifically (Table 2 Appendix C). Individual studies of people with neck pain were only included when there was no available evidence from systematic reviews on WAD, or where a study was published more recently and was therefore not included in the original systematic review.

2.3.3 Inclusion criteria for studies

The criteria for selecting studies were:

- Studies that included people with WAD (acceleration/deceleration injuries) and gave separate results for this group

- Studies that compared interventions carried out by physiotherapists with each other or with a control group receiving standard treatment, no treatment, or a placebo or sham procedure

- Randomised or controlled clinical trials have been reviewed where these are available

- Studies that included adult study participants only

- Where specific information for people with whiplash injuries was not available then systematic reviews and studies that included only people with neck (cervical spine) pain, and not people with neck and/or shoulder or back pain, were considered

- English language papers, as resources were not available for translation.

2.3.4 Final update search

The final update search was the most comprehensive search that was carried out and captured over a thousand citations. After sifting through the titles and abstracts, 16 references were found to be relevant to the therapy section of the guidelines (sections 4.1–4.3). 11 of the 16 studies and systematic reviews were discarded because they:

- Were discussion papers, letters or commentaries of studies[16, 17-19]

- Were already included in the review, either individually or as part of a systematic review[20–22]

- Were not randomised controlled trials [23–25]

- Included a report of methods used in a study, but included no results.[26]

Five studies matched the inclusion criteria and were obtained for further examination.[27–31] Of these:

- In one paper, people with WAD were excluded from the study[28]

- In one paper manipulation techniques were compared but the guiedelines' specific clinical questions were not addressed[31]

- In one paper an intervention that is not commonly used by physiotherapists was investigated[30]

- Two papers were updates of studies already included in the review section of the guidelines and the results have been added.[27, 29]

The references found were imported into bibliographic software (Reference Manager, EndNote) where possible and duplicates eliminated. The first stage of reviewing involved sifting through the EndNote database and identifying references that did not fit the inclusion criteria based on their titles alone. The next stage of elimination involved looking at the abstracts of the remaining references. The searches up to July 2002 yielded 1,016 unique references. After sifting through the references by title and abstract, 84 papers were obtained, and those which met the inclusion criteria were assessed in more detail.

From the 84 papers obtained, only 13 met all the inclusion criteria and were included in the evidence review.[32-44] One of these papers[37] was later excluded after discussion with the GDG as the intervention, ultra reiz current, was not thought by the expert group to be used by physiotherapists.

Data extraction forms for systematic reviews and studies were developed to enable pertinent information to be recorded and to assess the quality of the study or systematic review. A data extraction form was completed for each paper obtained and stored electronically .

Information extracted from the papers was entered into summary evidence tables describing briefly the patient groups, interventions and quality and giving the most relevant results of the studies included (Appendix C). The summaries of the evidence in sections 4.1–4.3 were then written, based on the evidence tables and in most cases without the need to go back to the original study reports. Elements of the study design and reporting that may have affected the reliability and accuracy of the results were highlighted and commented on in the text of the review and briefly in the summary tables.

2.4.1   Assessment of methodological quality

The randomised and controlled clinical trials were assessed for methodological quality using the same criteria as that used for the Physiotherapy Evidence Database (PEDro), see table 2.1.[45] This scale is based on a quality assessment tool developed by Delphi consensus (The Delphi List) by Verhagen et al.[46]

Table 2.1 The PEDro Scale[45]

1	Eligibility criteria were specified (assesses external validity – not included in final score)	No / Yes
2	Subjects were randomly allocated to groups (in a crossover study, subjects were randomly allocated an order in which treatments were received)	No / Yes
3	Allocation was concealed	No / Yes
4	The groups were similar at baseline regarding the most important prognostic indicators	No / Yes
5	There was blinding of all subjects	No / Yes
6	There was blinding of all therapists who administered the therapy	No / Yes
7	There was blinding of all assessors who measured at least one key outcome	No / Yes
8	Measures of at least one key outcome were obtained from more than 85% of the subjects initially allocated to groups	No / Yes
9	All subjects for whom outcome measures were available received the treatment or control condition as allocated or, where this was not the case, data for at least one key outcome was analysed by 'intention to treat'	No / Yes
10	The results of between-group statistical comparisons are reported for at least one key outcome	No / Yes
11	The study provides both point measures and measures of variability for at least one key outcome	No / Yes

The reviewer carried out a quality assessment of the included studies. Scores were compared with those on the PEDro website to minimise possible bias. For studies where the two scores differed, another member of the GDG was asked to assess the quality of the studies in question to settle the disagreement. The producers of PEDro were notified of any discrepancies between the scores allocated in this review and those in their database. Therefore, PEDro scores given for studies in the evidence review and the evidence tables in Appendix C, Table 1 are those allocated for these guidelines and may not be the same as the scores shown on the PEDro website. PEDro scores have been found to be reliable for use in systematic reviews.[47]

A decision was made by the GDG that studies receiving scores of five out of ten and above were judged as high quality and those with four out of ten or less were low quality. Of the 11 studies included in this evidence review, six[32,33,35,38-40,42] were considered as high quality and five[34,36,41,43,44] were low quality.

All factors in the PEDro scale are important features of a controlled clinical trial and items in the PEDro scale are given equal weight. However, some elements could potentially bias the results of the studies more than others.

The following factors were considered to be most significant to this review:

- Whether participants were randomised to groups

- If the outcome measurements had been carried out without knowledge of the group allocation

- The proportion of participants who withdrew from the study

- If an intention-to-treat analysis was used.

It is important to bear in mind that some of the items in the PEDro score may not be achievable in many physiotherapy clinical trials. In particular, blinding of therapists and patients is impossible in a large number of trials unless it is feasible for the control group to receive a placebo or sham procedure. Only one of the included studies was able to blind participants and therapists by using a pulsed electromagnetic therapy unit versus a dummy unit made by the manufacturer to look exactly the same.[35] The remaining studies were not able to use blinding because of the nature of the interventions compared, and therefore could not achieve maximum scores regardless of the way in which the studies might have been conducted.

The PEDro scores were therefore used as a guide to the overall quality of the studies included in the review. However, other aspects of the included studies that are not included in the PEDro scale were also considered in drawing up guidelines for clinical practice, for example, the length of follow up in the study. An intervention might be more effective in the short-term, but could be equally as effective as another treatment after a longer time period.

2.4.2 Levels of evidence

An evidence summary (ES) is provided at the end of each section of the evidence review, with an indication of the level of the evidence summarised. The levels of evidence used (Table 2.2) are those recommended in the CSP Information Paper 'Guidance for Developing Clinical Guidelines'.[48]

Table 2.2 Levels of evidence (adapted from CSP)[48]

Level	Type of evidence
Ia	Evidence obtained from a systematic review of randomised controlled trials
Ib	Evidence obtained from at least one randomised controlled trial
IIa	Evidence obtained from at least one well-designed controlled study without randomisation or a poor quality RCT
IIb	Evidence obtained from at least one other type of well-designed quasi-experimental study
III	Evidence obtained from well-designed non-experimental descriptive studies, such as comparative studies, correlation studies and case studies
IV	Evidence obtained from expert committee reports or opinions and/or clinical experience of respected authorities e.g. from the Delphi questionnaire

Study design is therefore used to indicate the extent to which results are reliable and robust. However, in these guidelines, levels of evidence do not take account of possible methodological flaws that may jeopardise the reliability of the results. Therefore evidence derived from poor quality RCTs and from RCTs with serious methodological flaws was down graded by one level compared to evidence from good quality RCTs. Where evidence was found for non-specific neck pain (in the absence of evidence for whiplash injury), the level of evidence is given, but the GDG also sought consensus views using the Delphi process. Methodological quality issues, particularly those thought to have the most influence on results, were considered alongside the levels of evidence when the recommendations for clinical practice were written.

2.5 Consensus development

2.5.1 Choosing the method

At the first meeting of the GDG it was recognised that the literature relating to WAD would be incomplete and inconsistent. Four methods of reaching consensus were considered (Table 2.3).

Table 2.3 Methods of reaching a consensus (adapted from Heath Technology Assessment)[49]

Consensus Method	Comment
Informal methods	The GDG could come to an informal consensus in an internal meeting
The Delphi technique	A wider reference group of experts would be selected and asked to complete a questionnaire to give their opinion on the points that needed agreement. More than one round of questionnaires could be used in an effort to move towards consensus
The Nominal Group Technique	Discussion within the group followed by voting in an iterative process leading to a group judgement
A Consensus Development Conference	A representative group is brought together to listen to the evidence before retiring to consider the questions and reach a judgement

It was unanimously agreed to use the Delphi technique where possible. Informal methods were not the first choice because they lack the scientific credibility that makes the process of reaching consensus transparent. Funds were not available to run a consensus development conference and it was agreed that it would be important to aim to include a wider group than would be included in a nominal group. However, where issues arose after the Delphi questionnaire was finalised the GDG was used as an expert consensus group, discussing the issue in question until they were able to agree a response/conclusion.

2.5.2 The Delphi technique

The Delphi technique was initially developed at the RAND Corporation during the 1950s and 1960s as a structured process for gathering knowledge from a panel of experts using a series of questionnaires with controlled feedback of opinion. Delphi was used to predict future trends but it has increasingly been used to gather research information on opinion about public health and educational issues.[50,51]

Delphi methods are designed to circumvent some of the disadvantages of traditional 'expert panels' as each Delphi panel member responds individually to the questionnaires. Thus there is no need for meetings, costs are reduced and group dynamics inhibiting less vocal participants are avoided. Anonymity is assured because panel members are never identified with their opinions and peer pressure or political awkwardness is avoided. For example, a panellist may have an opinion that is shared by few other panel members, but she or he is perfectly free to maintain that opinion, even when aware that the majority opinion differs. Delphi sees consensus as data, not as a goal. Though there have been critics of Delphi methods as a research tool, their criticisms have mostly been directed at assumptions of hard predictive value;[49,52] Delphi studies are generally accepted as appropriate tools for seeking opinion.

2.5.3 Practical details of the Delphi Methods

Gaps and inconsistencies in the evidence were apparent once the review of the literature was complete; the GDG members highlighted gaps in background literature. From these the first round of the Delphi questionnaire (Appendix D) was drafted, revised and piloted before being distributed to physiotherapists in early September 2003. The majority of questions involved assessing a statement on a five point Likert scale. A total of 68 Delphi questionnaires were sent to a range of physiotherapists working at different grades and in different clinical settings (Appendix F) and two reminders were sent to non-responders. In total 39 (57%) were returned completed. In view of the length of the questionnaire (128 statements, three open questions and three questions relating to personal details) the response rate for a postal questionnaire was considered good.

Questionnaires were returned by early October 2003 and data were transferred manually to an Excel spreadsheet. Data were entered twice, the two spreadsheets compared and errors corrected. The open questions were analysed i.e. recommended textbooks for assessment of WAD, barriers to recovery and suggested outcome measures. This added 20 additional statements to the second round of the Delphi questionnaire which contained no open questions. The extent to which physiotherapists had agreed with each statement on the first round was calculated and displayed on the questionnaire in the second round (Appendix E).

The second round of the Delphi questionnaire was sent out in late October and returned by mid December 2003. Once again two reminders were sent and results were analysed as in the first round to give a final score for each question. Questionnaires were sent to the 39 physiotherapists who responded to the first round and 27 (69%) were returned.

There is no standard threshold for consensus. A decision from the GDG was therefore necessary to determine the definition of consensus for these guidelines. In previous health care studies consensus has been set at 51%,[53] 66%[54] and 75%.[55] Having read the literature and consulted with experts in Delphi methods, the GDG met in March 2004 and agreed on the following definitions: *majority view* (over half of the participants in agreement), *consensus* (three-quaters or more in agreement) and *unanimity* (all in agreement).

Table 2.4 Definitions of agreement from the results of the Delphi questionnaire

Percent of respondents	Definition of agreement
100%	Unanimity
75–99 %	Consensus
51–74%	Majority view
0–50%	No consensus

The percentages used to categorise the level of consensus agreement were derived by combining data for 'strongly agree' and 'agree', and again combining 'strongly disagree' and 'disagree' from the second Delphi round questionnaires, and calculating these as a percentage of the total data for that question. These percentage figures are set out in Appendix G and are used throughout sections three and four, where the results of the Delphi process are discussed.

2.6 Developing recommendations for practice

Guideline writing involves bridging the gap between theory and practice i.e. moving from the evidence (research, consensus and expert opinion) to the formulation of recommendations based on the interpretation of the evidence in relation to clinical practice. The GDG took account of this when they met to agree on the recommendations. There were three levels of interpretation as follows:

- A **direct link between the Delphi results and the recommendations**; the Delphi questions were designed for this purpose

- An **interpretation of the research evidence on physiotherapy interventions, from which recommendations were derived** (sections 4.1 to 4.3); the link was fairly clear where studies related to physiotherapy practice

- A **logical link from the research evidence/expert opinion in the supporting sections** (all sections except 4.1 to 4.3) **to recommendations**; the studies and literature used were often not directly related to physiotherapy and hence more interpretation was necessary to tease out relevant issues.

2.7 Grading the Recommendations

The recommendations for practice are derived from the literature and from the Delphi questionnaire. Each recommendation is graded according to the type of evidence on which it was based (Table 2.5).

Table 2.5 Grading guidelines recommendations (adapted from CSP)[48]

Grade	Evidence
A	At least one randomised controlled trial of overall good quality and consistency addressing the specific recommendation (evidence levels Ia and Ib in Table 2.2)
B	Well-conducted clinical studies but no randomised clinical trials on the topic of the recommendation (evidence levels IIa, IIb and III in Table 2.2)
C	Evidence from Delphi methods or other expert committee reports. This indicates that directly applicable clinical studies of good quality are absent (evidence level IV in Table 2.2)
Good practice point	Recommended good practice based on the clinical experience of the GDG

Few grade **A** recommendations are made in this document because there have been few randomised controlled trials in this field. The result is heavy reliance on consensus evidence and hence many grade **C** recommendations. However some issues arose after the Delphi questionnaire had been finalised and these gaps were addressed by the GDG arriving at a consensus i.e. by informal methods. This led to the **good practice points** that are the least reliable of the recommendations. Guidelines development is an ongoing and iterative process and these issues will be considered for any future Delphi questionnaire for the next edition of this document planned for 2010.

The recommendations that follow in sections 4.1–4.3 are based on established methods and involved a systematic review of the literature and consensus seeking where evidence was incomplete or contradictory. Each recommendation is clearly graded to indicate the strength of evidence on which it is based. The recommendations relating to section 3 and sections 4.4, 4.5 provide background information and highlight links to other literature that are likely to be of use to physiotherapists and people with WAD. However, these were not subject to a full systematic review, as was carried out for sections 4.1–4.3.

2.8 Referencing style

The Vancouver referencing system is used throughout these guidelines i.e. references are numbered in the order that they appear in the text and listed in this order at the end of the guidelines (section 14). This method was chosen as it is a widely used and accepted method of referencing and so that lists of authors' names do not interfere with the readability of the document. However, to ensure the references are accessible they are also presented alphabetically in Appendix M.

2.9 Cost and safety of interventions

Although the GDG intended to address the issues of cost and safety of interventions this was not possible due to the paucity of literature in these areas. Details of risks of treatments are given where information is available e.g. the adverse events from cervical manipulation in section 4.2.2.

2.10 AGREE instrument

The GDG referred regularly to the AGREE Instrument[56] during the production of these guidelines to ensure that a structured and rigorous methodology was followed.

Physiotherapy assessment and associated issues

In 1928 'whiplash' was first introduced as a term for an injury to the neck due to rapid acceleration-deceleration forces on the upper spine.[57] This most commonly happens in a motor vehicle accident when a stationary vehicle is hit from the rear. Until recently it was thought that firstly the head and neck were forced into hyperextension, with horizontal translation as the head lagged behind the movement of the torso. Secondly, the head and neck overcame the resulting inertia and became hyperflexed. Thus tissues in the cervical spine were put under great stress as they were compressed or stretched, to cause injury.

However a new theory, based upon biomechanical studies, has given a possible explanation of the forces acting on the spine. The theory, which is based on in vivo and in vitro whiplash simulations, accepts that the force arises from a rear impact but suggests that the C6 vertebrae initially rotates backward into extension before any upper cervical movement occurs. As C6 reaches maximum extension C5 is forced to extend. The result is an S-shaped curve[58] with the lower cervical vertebrae in extension and the upper cervical spine in relative flexion. Alternatively the mechanism may be bi-phasic with the S-shaped curve in the first phase leading to a second phase where all levels of the spine hyperextend, creating a C shaped curve. The cervical spine is forced into these positions in less than 200ms.[59] The result is that the most affected level of the spine is at C5/C6 with disc disruption, stretching of capsular ligaments and facet trauma. There is maximal elongation of the C6/C7 level and the vertebral artery during the S-shaped position.[59] The S-shaped position causes shear movement at the upper cervical spine which may lead to upper cervical pain and headaches.[60] It has been suggested that the cervical spine as a whole does not exceed its normal physiological limits although the lower cervical levels do exceed limits of segmental posterior rotation, resulting in the posterior articular processes impacting and anterior separation.[61]

A recent study concluded that the lower cervical spine is at risk of extension injury in both the S and C phase but the upper cervical spine is at risk of extension injury at higher impact only. Flexion injury was found to be less likely.[58, 62]

Evidence Summary 1	Level
The mechanisms of whiplash injury	
• The mechanisms of injury may indicate the cervical level affected	IIb
• Mechanisms of injury are not yet fully understood, but theories are being developed	IIb

Recommendations (ES 1)	Grade
Physiotherapists should be aware of theories that are developing to explain the mechanism of whiplash injury in order that they can relate the site of injury to the person's symptoms and plan their physiotherapy management.	B

The Quebec Classification[2] and a new Swedish classification based on functional impairment and disability[63] have both been considered as part of the guidelines development process. The Quebec Classification was unanimously chosen by the GDG as the most clinically useful tool for physiotherapists with its clear definition of minimal injury, more major problems and serious injury. However, Hartling et al suggested that grade II in the original Quebec Classification should be subdivided into II a and II b to distinguish between people with normal range of movement and those with limited range of movement.[64] This is important because the latter group have greater risk of a poor prognosis.

Table 3.1 Clinical classification of whiplash associated disorders.

Adapted from Spitzer et al[2] and Hartling[64]

WAD Grade	Clinical Presentation
O	No neck complaint No physical sign(s)
I	Neck complaint of pain, stiffness or merely tenderness No physical sign(s)

II	Neck complaint and musculoskeletal sign(s) *
	A retrospective cohort study[64] has suggested further classification of grade II WAD:
	    II a point tenderness and normal range of movement
	    II b point tenderness and limited range of movement
	          (greater risk of long term symptoms)

III	Neck complaint and neurological sign(s) * *
IV	Neck complaint and fracture or dislocation
*	Musculoskeletal signs include decreased range of motion and point tenderness
* *	Neurological signs include decreased or absent deep tendon reflexes, weakness and sensory deficits.

Evidence summary 2	Level
The Quebec classification appears to be the most clinically useful system available for the classification of WAD	IV

Recommendations (ES 2)	Grade
The Quebec Task Force classification should be used by physiotherapists for WAD with grade II subdivided into IIa and IIb, in order to assist with diagnosis and prognosis.	Good practice point

3.3 Recovery

3.3.1 Pain

Several studies have considered the prevalence and prognosis for people with WAD in terms of pain.

US insurance company data[65] suggests that:

- A third of car occupants involved in an accident experience neck pain (33%)

- A third of these attend emergency health services (11%)

- A third of these consult their primary care practitioner (3%)

- A third of these consult more than once (1%)

- A third of these develop chronic WAD (0.33%).

This suggests that 1 in 300 people involved in a car crash develop chronic pain.[65] These data are summarised in figure 3.1.

Figure 3.1 Bar chart illustrating prevelance of people with WAD developing chronic pain

(US insurance company data)[65]

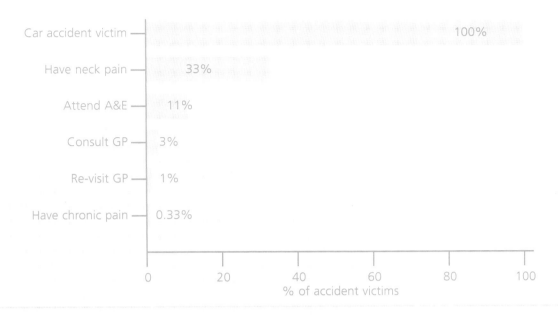

Data from US hospitals for people with WAD suggest that:

- 60% report that symptoms subside after one month and that they are pain free after three months
- 75% have recovered from symptoms after six months
- 85% have recovered after three years
- 15% continue to report symptoms after three years

Figure 3.2 Line graph illustrating percentage of people experiencing neck pain over time

(US hospital data)[66]

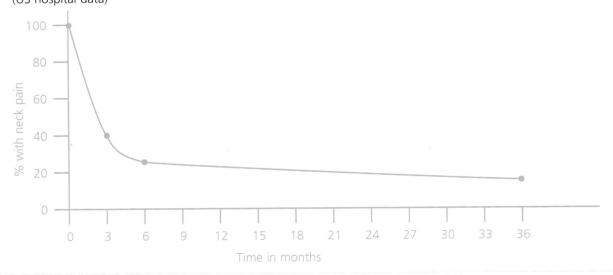

This data also suggests that severe pain is reported by 4% of people with WAD after 3 years.[66]

A proportion of people with WAD have or complain of symptoms for much longer than it takes their tissues to heal. 6–18% of people with WAD may have significant symptoms up to two years after injury.[67,68] But the prognosis for people who consult with persistent symptoms at six months is reasonably optimistic. Analysis of studies with long term follow-up (3–10 years), suggests that of those with chronic symptoms (6 months duration):

- 40% are still likely to recover

- 44% are likely to report some residual symptoms (i.e. mild to moderate)

- 16% are likely to be left with severe symptoms.[66,69]

3.3.2 Quality of life

WAD may reduce quality of life. A long term study (n=104) using the Sickness Impact Profile demonstrated lower than average mood and function two and a half years after whiplash injury.[70]

3.3.3 Psychological factors

Anxiety and depression may be prevalent in people with WAD and may be more important in affecting cognitive function than physical factors or pain.[71] Following up people with WAD (previously seen at two and 10 years post injury) at 15 years post-injury (n=81) ongoing depression and anxiety was observed.[72]

3.3.4 Time taken to return to work

Canadian insurance data suggests that for those with WAD the average time taken to return to work is roughly one month after injury.[73] Irish health care records for those with chronic symptoms (greater than six months duration) suggest that on average people returned to work after nearly five months.[74]

3.3.5 The advice that should be given to people about recovery from WAD

Delphi findings indicate that it is good practice for physiotherapists to advise people with WAD that they are very likely to recover (*unanimity* 100%). Thus, in addition to the level III evidence that only a small proportion of people with WAD take longer than would be expected to recover, there is level IV evidence about the advice that should be given.

Evidence Summary 3	Level
The prognosis and natural history of WAD	
• A small proportion of people with WAD take longer than would be expected to recover	III
• There is *unanimity* (100%) that it is good practice for physiotherapists to advise people with WAD that they are very likely to recover	IV

Recommendations (ES 3)	Grade
Physiotherapists should advise people with WAD that they are very likely to recover.	C

3.4 Risk factors that may influence prognosis

This section considers the risk factors associated with WAD that may influence recovery following a whiplash injury. Prognostic factors include circumstances at the time of injury, factors that were present before injury and post-injury factors.

3.4.1 Circumstances at the time of injury

This section is applied specifically to motor vehicle accidents but similar questions should be considered in the case of sporting accidents.

There is conflicting evidence about the effect of a rear end collision. Some studies suggest that there is a greater risk of WAD when people are involved in rear end collisions; for example a UK prospective study (n=1197)[75] and a German retrospective study (n=1,096).[76] Nevertheless a systematic review of 50 reports on 29 cohorts of people concludes that rear end collision does not lead to a poor prognosis.[77]

Headrests should be correctly positioned i.e. level with the top of the head and close to the back of the head (no greater than 5 cm gap) if they are to reduce the incidence of neck trauma.[78] A specially designed seat to reduce loading on individual areas of the spine and absorb some of the impact has been developed.[79]

There is conflicting evidence on whether the speed of a collision is a predisposing factor for WAD. It seems logical that increased speed of impact should increase the risk of WAD, although a German study of computerised biomechanical analysis (n=1,096) of drivers involved in litigation indicates that low impact speeds (up to 20km/h) can result in WAD.[76]

Low weight or relatively low weight vehicles may be a risk factor for WAD:

- A German study of computerised biomechanical analysis (n=1096) of drivers involved in litigation indicates that drivers of lighter cars are more likely to sustain a whiplash injury; low speeds only were studied (up to 20km/h)[76]

- An Australian cohort study (n=246) collected data via telephone interviews and concluded that a heavy striking vehicle compared with the driver's vehicle led to increased incidence of whiplash.[80]

There is conflicting evidence on whether wearing a seat belt is a predisposing factor for WAD. Whilst the introduction of seatbelts has saved many from serious injury there is evidence that they may have increased the risk of WAD.[2,81-84] A population based study in the Netherlands did not find the incidence of seat belt use increased between 1989 and 1995,[85] yet there was an increase in neck sprain. This may have been due to an increased reporting of WAD, increased car usage, or increased number of vehicles on the roads.[85, 68]

Delphi findings suggest that the following indicate increased likelihood of severe symptoms:

- Poorly positioned headrest (consensus 88%)

- Looking to one side during a read-end collision (85%)

Thus, in addition to level III evidence, there is some level IV evidence that specific circumstances at the time of injury may affect prognosis.

Evidence Summary 4	Level
Risk factors at the time of injury	
• Low relative weight of vehicle that the person is travelling in	III
• Poorly positioned headrests	IV
• Rear end collisions when the person is looking to one side	IV

3.4.2 Pre existing factors affecting prognosis

Pre-existing factors can indicate that a poor prognosis is likely following injury. Research suggests that pre-trauma neck ache is an indicator of a poor prognosis following whiplash:

- A prospective epidemiological study in Sweden (n=296)[86]

- A prospective study in the UK (n=7,669)[87]

- A retrospective study in Australia (n=246)[80]

- A retrospective study in Lithuania (n=202).[88]

There was also *consensus* (96%) that pre-trauma neck ache indicates that a poor prognosis is likely following whiplash injury (Delphi finding).

Research findings are inconsistent about whether a particular age group is more likely to experience a poor prognosis following whiplash. Nevertheless age has often been considered a risk factor.[2,13,46,75,80,89,90] There is evidence, from a systematic review of 50 papers reporting on 29 prospective cohort studies, that older age is not associated with adverse prognosis for recovery from WAD.[77]

At the same time, retrospective epidemiological studies suggest that the highest incidence age groups may be:

- 20–24 year olds followed by 25–34 year olds[2]

- 25–54 year old[90]

- 25–29 year olds (a 25 year study of people attending the accident and emergency department of a Netherlands' hospital n=694).[91]

Furthermore, a prospective study of people with WAD attending an accident and emergency department in the UK (n=1,197) suggests that the highest incidence age group is:

- 40–49 year olds followed by 30–39 year olds.[75]

The variation in results may be a result of the use of different research methodologies, national variations or different data collection settings i.e. hospital or insurance records.

Many epidemiological studies suggest that being female is a significant risk factor for developing symptoms of WAD.[2, 75, 80, 85, 92–94] Despite this a systematic review of 50 studies reporting on 29 prospective cohort studies reported strong evidence that female gender did not affect prognosis for recovery from WAD.[77] There was no consensus on this (Delphi finding).

There was *consensus* (93%) that pre-existing degenerative changes indicate that a poor prognosis is likely following whiplash injury (Delphi finding). There was a *majority view* (59%) that a history of pre-trauma headache indicates that a poor prognosis is likely following whiplash injury (Delphi finding).

There was *consensus* (85%) that a low level of job satisfaction indicates that a poor prognosis is likely following whiplash injury (Delphi finding).

To summarise the Delphi findings on the effect of pre-existing factors on WAD, the following indicate that a poor prognosis is likely:

- Pre-trauma neck ache (consensus 96%)

- Pre-existing degenerative changes (consensus 93%)

- Low level of job satisfaction (consensus 85%)

- Pre-trauma headaches (majority view 59%)

There was no agreement in the Delphi findings that people below 50 years old or females were likely to have a poor prognosis.

Thus in addition to the level III evidence, there is some level IV evidence that pre-existing factors may led to a poor prognosis.

Evidence Summary 5	Level
Pre-existing risk factors may include	
• Pre-trauma neck ache	III
• Pre-existing degenerative changes (consensus 93%)	IV
• Low level of job satisfaction (consensus 85%)	IV
• Pre-trauma headaches (majority view 59%)	IV
• Evidence is conflicting about whether age or gender is a risk factor	III

3.4.3 Post-injury factors influencing prognosis

A systematic review of prospective cohort studies (n=29) found strong evidence that high initial pain intensity tends to lead to a slower recovery of function.[77]

Delphi findings indicate that the following post-injury factors suggest a poor prognosis is likely following WAD:

- Headache for more than six months following injury (*consensus* (96%)
- Neurological signs present after injury (*consensus* 93%)

Evidence Summary 6	Level
Post-injury risk factors may include	
• High initial pain intensity	III
• Headache for more than six months following injury (*consensus* 96%)	IV
• Neurological signs present after injury (*consensus* 93%)	IV

Recommendations	Grade
Risk factors	
Information should be sought in order that risk factors can be identified at the assessment stage as they can adversely affect prognosis.	
At the time of injury, the following factors indicate that a poorer prognosis is likely (ES 4)	
• Relatively low weight of person's vehicle compared with other vehicle involved	B
• Poor headrest position (i.e. not level with the top of the head, not close to the back of the head)	C
• Rear end collisions where the person is looking to one side.	C
The following pre-existing factors indicate that a poorer prognosis is likely (ES 5)	
• Pre-trauma neck ache	B
• Pre-existing degenerative changes	C
• Low level of job satisfaction	C
• Pre-trauma headaches	C
The following post-injury factors indicate that a poorer prognosis is likely (ES 6)	
• High initial pain intensity	B
• Headache for more than six months following injury	C
• Neurological signs present after injury	C

3.4.4 Psychosocial barriers to recovery

Pathology-based medical models assume a strong relationship exists between physical abnormality, pain and disability. However, research conducted with people who report chronic pain has shown that there is often only a weak association between these factors.[95] In light of this, alternative theories have been proposed as a means of explaining why some people adjust relatively well to chronic pain whilst others do not. Studies suggest that adjustment to chronic pain is strongly related to psychosocial as well as biomedical factors.[95-97] Furthermore, psychosocial factors appear to be better predictors of work absence than either biomedical or ergonomic factors.[96-100]

This section considers what have been described as yellow flags i.e. the psychological and sociological barriers to recovery from WAD, and the stage at which these should be assessed. The New Zealand Acute Low Back Pain Guidelines identify a number of yellow flags associated with chronicity.[101] Although the New Zealand guidelines do not relate specifically to whiplash or cervical spine injury, it is possible that many of the factors identified will also affect recovery in WAD. A number of these yellow flags are listed below. Sections 3.4.4.1 to 3.4.4.8 are based on the work of Waddell (1998)[102] and

Kendall et al (1997)[101] except where referenced to another author.

It is important that these factors be assessed, and where appropriate targeted for change, when treating people with WAD.

3.4.4.1 Attitudes and beliefs about pain

Examples of attitudes and beliefs about pain that can be considered psychosocial barriers to recovery:

- Belief that pain is harmful
- Belief that pain must be completely abolished before attempting to return to work or normal activity
- Belief that pain is uncontrollable
- Catastrophising (i.e. thinking the worst; misinterpreting bodily sensations).

3.4.4.2 Behaviours of people with WAD towards pain

Examples of behaviours towards pain that may signal an increased likelihood of psychosocial barriers:

- Use of extended rest
- Reduced activity level with significant withdrawal from activities of daily living
- Report of extremely high pain intensity e.g. around 10 on a 0–10 visual analogue scale.

3.4.4.3 Clinician behaviours

Examples of clinician reinforcing yellow flags:

- Health professional sanctioning disability; not providing interventions that will improve function
- Diagnostic language leading to catastrophising and fear (e.g. fear of long term damage)
- Dramatisation of WAD by health professional producing dependency on treatments, and continuation of passive treatment
- Expectation of a 'techno-fix' i.e. that the body can be 'fixed' like a machine.

3.4.4.4 Compensation issues

Examples of compensation issues that may have a negative impact on recovery:

- Lack of financial incentive to return to work
- History of extended time off work due to injury or other pain problem (e.g. more than 12 weeks).

Literature regarding the effect of litigation on WAD reaches a range of conclusions. A prospective study (n=39) suggested that the health status of people with WAD often improves with treatment despite pending litigation.[103] In addition, a retrospective study (n=102) involving a two year follow up[104] and another longitudinal study (n=100) indicate that settlement of compensation does not appear to be followed by any marked improvement in clinical state.[104,105] Furthermore a systematic review of 50 reports on 29 prospective cohort studies reported strong evidence that compensation is not associated with an adverse prognosis.[77] A systematic review of 13 cohort studies concluded that recovery was faster in countries where litigation is less common.[106]

In view of the range of conclusions drawn from the research findings, a question was posed as part of the Delphi process. Delphi findings indicate that unresolved legal issues suggest that a poor prognosis is likely following WAD (*consensus* 81%). However, it was felt the research and Delphi evidence was sufficiently uncertain for only a tentative recommendation to be made.

3.4.4.5 Emotions of people with WAD that could hinder recovery

Examples of emotions influencing WAD are:

- Fear of increased pain with activity or work

- Depression, loss of sense of enjoyment

- Feeling useless and not needed

- Anxiety about and heightened awareness of body sensations

- More irritability than usual.

3.4.4.6 Post-traumatic stress reaction

A prospective study found people with whiplash injury (n=76) were psychologically distressed but that as symptoms subsided the stress was reduced. Those with moderate to severe symptoms at six months post-injury tended to have moderate post-traumatic stress reaction.[107]

3.4.4.7 Family

Examples of family issues that may hinder recovery are:

- Over protective partner/spouse, emphasising fear of harm or encouraging catastrophising (usually well intentioned)

- Solicitous behaviour from spouse (e.g. taking over tasks).

3.4.4.8 Work

Examples of work factors are:

- Belief that work is harmful; that it will do damage or be dangerous

- Unsupportive or unhappy current work environment

- Job involves significant biomechanical demands such as lifting, manual handling of heavy items, driving, vibration.

Delphi findings indicate that the following may be barriers to recovery from WAD:

- High fear of pain and movement (fear that pain and/or movement leads to harm) (*unanimity* 100%)

- Low self-efficacy (lacking confidence in ability to undertake a particular activity (*unanimity* 100%)

- Severe anxiety (*unanimity* 100%)

- Evidence of severe depression (*unanimity* 100%)

- Low pain locus of control (believing that it is impossible to control the pain) (*unanimity* 100%)

- High use of passive coping strategies (withdrawal/passing on responsibility for pain controls to others) (*unanimity* 100%)

- Chronic widespread pain (*consensus* 96%)

- High tendency to catastrophise (*consensus* 96%)

- Problems in relationships with others (*consensus* 92%)

- A series of previously failed treatments (*consensus* 92%)

- Non compliance with treatment and advice (*consensus* 88%)

- Unrealistic expectations of treatment (*consensus* 86%)

- Inability to work because of the pain (*consensus* 85%)

- Negative expectations of treatment (*consensus* 81%)

- Poor understanding of the healing mechanism (*consensus* 80%)

- Failure of the physiotherapist to address an individual person's needs (*consensus* 80%)

- Poor clinical reasoning by the physiotherapist (*consensus* 69%).

Delphi findings indicate that the barriers to recovery should be assessed at the following stages after injury:

after 6 weeks and before 12 weeks (*consensus* 85%)
at 12 weeks or more (*consensus* 82%)
after 2 weeks and before 6 weeks (*consensus* 81%)
less than 2 weeks after injury (*majority view* 56%).

Evidence Summary 7	Level
Psychosocial barriers to recovery from WAD (yellow flags)	
Psychosocial factors, as barriers to recovery, may be associated with attitudes and beliefs about pain, behaviours, compensation issues, clinician behaviours, emotions, family and work.	IV
The following may be barriers to recovery from WAD:	
• High fear of pain and movement (*unanimity* 100%)	IV
• Low self-efficacy (*unanimity* 100%)	IV
• Severe anxiety (*unanimity* 100%)	IV
• Severe depression (*unanimity* 100%)	IV
• Low pain locus of control (*unanimity* 100%)	IV
• High use of passive coping strategies (*unanimity* 100%)	IV
• Chronic widespread pain (*consensus* 96%)	IV
• High tendency to catastrophise (*consensus* 96%)	IV
• Problems in relationships with others (*consensus* 92%)	IV
• A series of previously failed treatments (*consensus* 92%)	IV
• Non-compliance with treatment and advice (*consensus* 88%)	IV
• Unrealistic expectations of treatment (*consensus* 86%)	IV
• Inability to work because of the pain (*consensus* 85%)	IV
• Negative expectations of treatment (*consensus* 81%)	IV
• Poor understanding of the healing mechanism (*consensus* 80%)	IV
• Failure of the physiotherapist to meet an individual person's needs (*consensus* 80%)	IV
• Poor clinical reasoning by the physiotherapist (*majority view* 69%)	IV
Compensation issues do not appear to affect prognosis.	III
People with moderate to severe symptoms at six months post-injury are likely to experience a moderate post-traumatic stress reaction.	III
Barriers to recovery should be considered:	
• After 6 weeks and before 12 weeks (*consensus* 85%)	IV
• At 12 weeks or more (*consensus* 82%)	IV
• After 2 weeks and before 6 weeks (*consensus* 81%)	IV
• Less than 2 weeks after injury (*majority view* 56%).	IV

3.4.5 Occupational barriers to recovery

Recent work suggests that there are types of occupational risk factors, described as blue and black flags.[108] These are:

- blue flags are perceived barriers to return to work e.g. perceived inadequate support from managers, perceived time pressures
- black flags are the actual barriers to return to work e.g. the benefit system or sickness policy make return to work a less desirable course of action.

A reference to blue and black flags is included for completeness. At the time of writing, the GDG did not feel that physiotherapists generally use blue and black flags in practice and these are not therefore discussed in detail.

Evidence Summary 8	Level
Occupational barriers to recovery (blue and black flags) may include	
• Perceptions of work e.g. high demand and low control, perceived time pressure	IV
• Job context and working conditions	IV

Recommendations	Grade
Barriers to recovery	
Psychosocial barriers to recovery (ES 7)	
• Compensation issues may not be a barrier to recovery from WAD	B
• Physiotherapists should be aware of the wide range of psychosocial barriers to recovery:	C

- · high fear of pain and movement
- · low self-efficacy
- · severe anxiety
- · severe depression
- · low pain locus of control
- · high use of passive coping strategies
- · chronic widespread pain
- · high tendency to catastrophise
- · problems in relationships with others
- · a series of previously failed treatments
- · non-compliance with treatment and advice
- · unrealistic expectations of treatment
- · inability to work because of the pain
- · negative expectations of treatment
- · poor understanding of the healing mechanism
- · failure of the physiotherapist to meet an individual person's needs
- · poor clinical reasoning by the physiotherapist

• Physiotherapists should assess for psychosocial barriers at all stages after injury	C
• Ongoing moderate to severe symptoms six months after injury are likely to be associated with post-traumatic stress syndrome.	C

Occupational barriers to recovery (ES 8)

Physiotherapists should be aware that perception of work and job context and working conditions may be barriers to recovery.	C

A wide range of symptoms are documented in association with WAD although many people with WAD will experience only neck, head and shoulder discomfort and are not affected by the more unusual symptoms.

3.5.1 Neck pain

Neck pain is the most commonly reported symptom of WAD.[109,110] Furthermore specific segmental zygapophyseal joint blocks have demonstrated that the neck and surrounding tissues are the most common source of chronic pain for people with WAD.[111,112] A prospective study (n=380) of people involved in a rear end motor vehicle accident found the most commonly reported symptom was neck pain, followed by headache, neck stiffness, low back pain, upper limb symptoms, dizziness, nausea and visual problems.[109] Tinnitus, temporomandibular joint pain, paraesthesia and concentration or memory disturbance may also be experienced.[110]

3.5.2 Headache

Headache is the second most common symptom, often in the sub-occipital region with referral to the temporal area. These areas are innervated from the upper cervical levels and it was found[112] that 50% of people complaining of headaches had pain arising from the C2/C3 segmental level.

3.5.3 Radiating pains to the head, shoulder, arms or interscapular area

Radiating pains to the head, shoulder, arms or interscapular area are often reported at some time post-injury. These patterns of somatic referral do not necessarily indicate which structure is the primary source of the pain but rather suggest the segmental level mediating nocioception.

3.5.4 Generalised hypersensitivity

Studies of small groups of people with WAD from Denmark (n=11)[113] and from Switzerland (n=27 and n=14)[114, 115] found that the people with WAD had generalised hypersensitivity, extending as far as the lower limbs, when compared with healthy volunteers. It was suggested that WAD might lead to spinal cord hyperexcitability causing exaggerated pain on peripheral stimulation.

3.5.5 Paraesthesia and muscle weakness

Paraesthesia and muscle weakness may be caused by cervical radiculopathy, thoracic outlet syndrome and spinal cord compression.[116]

3.5.6 Symptoms from the temporomandibular joint

Symptoms from the temporomandibular joint have been reported in the literature related to WAD but a study carried out in Lithuania[117] found only a 2.4% prevalence in 165 cases.

3.5.7 Visual disturbances

Visual disturbances are mentioned in the literature.[109,118,119] The pathophysiological basis for these symptoms has not been clearly established although a sympathetic nervous system link is possible.

3.5.8 Proprioceptive control of head and neck position

Although one study (n=27) found proprioceptive control of head and neck position reduced in 62% of people after whiplash injury the sample size was too small to draw general conclusions.[120]

3.5.9 Impaired cognitive function

Cognitive function may be impaired by WAD but there is some evidence that such symptoms may be as a result of chronic pain, chronic fatigue or depression.[121]

Evidence Summary 9	Level
The symptoms of WAD	
Many people with WAD experience neck, head and shoulder discomfort. However, a wide range of other symptoms may also be experienced	III

Recommendations (ES 9 and section 3.5)	Grade
Physiotherapists should be aware that the symptoms of WAD can include neck pain, headache, shoulder and arm pain, generalised hypersensitivity, paraesthesia and muscle weakness, temporomandibular joint pain and dysfunction, visual disturbance, impairment of the proprioceptive control of head and neck position and impaired cognitive function.	B

3.6 Assessment and examination

This section considers consent, entry into physiotherapy services, subjective assessment, serious pathology, psychological and occupational barriers to recovery, objective examination and the aims of physiotherapy intervention. The Delphi process sought consensus on textbooks that can provide a useful background to assessment. A list of these can be found in section 15.

3.6.1 Valid Consent

There is a legal and ethical principle that patients have a right to determine what happens to their bodies.[122] When people volunteer their consent, physiotherapists should establish that permission has been given to proceed with examination and treatment, and this should be recorded. Health professionals who do not respect an individual's autonomy may be disciplined by their employer and / or their professional organisation and sued through the civil courts. To give consent people must have the capacity to understand the nature, purpose and likely effects of treatment. They must be informed of substantial and relevant risks associated with proposed interventions. Physiotherapists should be familiar with the law on consent. They should follow CSP Core Standards 2005[123] and any local organisational policy and may contact the CSP for advice where necessary.

Evidence from a Department of Health guide also indicates responsibility for consent.[122]

Evidence Summary 10	Level
Valid Consent	
Valid consent must be sought prior to assessment and treatment	IV

3.6.2 Access to physiotherapy services

There is no single accepted way that people with WAD can access physiotherapy services. For this reason the Delphi questionnaire included a question seeking consensus firstly on how and secondly on who to prioritise into physiotherapy services.

Delphi findings indicate that, in the acute stage, entry to physiotherapy services is best prioritised by:

- A physiotherapist screening individual people (*consensus* 85%)
- A physiotherapist working in the accident and emergency department (*consensus* 78%)
- A physiotherapist assessing individual people by telephone (*majority view* 56%).

  Level

Entry into physiotherapy services in the acute stage should be prioritised by:

- A physiotherapist screening individual people (*consensus* 85%)   IV
- A physiotherapist working in the accident and emergency department (*consensus* 78%)   IV
- A physiotherapist assessing individual people by telephone (*majority view* 56%)   IV

At the point of entry there is another important decision to make when managing a busy service and that is which patients should be prioritised to enter the physiotherapy service?

Delphi findings indicate that the following factors make an individual person a higher priority at the assessment/screening stage:

- A person's activities of daily living are disrupted (*consensus* 96%)
- A person is off work (*consensus* 96%)
- The injury has occurred more recently (*consensus* 89%).

Evidence Summary 12   Level

The following people with WAD should be prioritised into the physiotherapy services:

- Those whose activities of daily living are disrupted (*consensus* 96%)   IV
- People off work (*consensus* 96%)   IV
- Those whose injury occurred more recently (*consensus* 89%)   IV

The GDG acknowledges that the questions relating to physiotherapy service provision might be expanded and improved in the future and that prioritisation must necessarily depend on local service provision.

3.6.3 Subjective assessment

Using their own clinical experience, the GDG developed this section through discussion and group consensus, to outline important issues at this stage of the assessment. It discusses understanding people's symptoms, the history of their presenting condition, past medical history, education and advice needs and their expectations of treatment.

3.6.3.1 Symptoms

People with WAD may present with any of the following symptoms: pain, paraesthesia, anaesthesia, stiffness, reduced function, visual disturbances and impaired cognitive function (section 3.5).

Assessment of symptoms should include:

- Site, including possible areas of referred pain i.e. neck pain, headaches, pain radiating into the head, shoulder, upper limbs or intrascapular area and temporomandibular joint
- Quality, frequency, depth and intensity
- Behaviour of the symptoms including the aggravating and easing factors and the 24-hour pattern of the symptoms
- Severity and irritability
- Links between the symptoms.

3.6.3.2 History of present condition

History of present condition should include:

- The mechanism of injury including details of the accident i.e. the speed, direction of impact, weight of the vehicle, use of seatbelt and head rest position, head position

- The onset of all the symptoms. These may include neck pain, headaches, pain radiating into the head, shoulder, upper limbs or intrascapular area, parasethesia, muscle weakness, temporomandibular involvement, visual disturbances, and impaired cognitive function

- Investigations made and the results of these

- Treatments given and their outcomes.

3.6.3.3 Past medical history

Subjective assessment should include:

- General health including previous major operations or illnesses (e.g. diabetes or epilepsy)

- Drugs taken e.g. steroids, anti-coagulants.

Evidence Summary 13	Level
Subjective assessment	
Subjective assessment involves identifying people's symptoms, the history of their presenting condition and their past medical history	IV

3.6.4 Serious pathology

3.6.4.1 Defining red flags

Red flags are defined as indicators of serious pathology. Unlike the red flag guidelines for low back pain,[124, 125] there are no published guidelines on red flags for whiplash or cervical spine injury. However there is some consensus on the signs and symptoms that should alert the clinician to the presence of potential serious pathology. The list below includes the range of signs and symptoms that should be treated as potential red flags. They have been divided into two categories i.e. those requiring immediate investigation via the nearest accident and emergency department and those that should be considered precautions to treatment.

3.6.4.2 Red flags

Symptoms needing urgent investigation if they develop after whiplash injury include:

- Bilateral paraesthesia in upper/lower limbs

- Gait disturbance e.g. tripping or coordination difficulty [126,127]

- Spastic paresis [126]

- Positive Lhermittes sign i.e. shooting pain or paraesthesia into lower limbs or all four limbs with cervical flexion

- Hyper reflexia [126]

- Nerve root signs at more than two adjacent levels [2,124,128]

- Progressively worsening neurological signs e.g. motor weakness, areflexia and sensory loss[2, 124, 125, 128]

- Symptoms of upper cervical instability[2, 129]

- Non-mechanical pain which is unremitting and severe.[124,125]

3.6.4.3 Precautions

Symptoms that should be seen as precautions to treatment include:

- Positive stress tests of the cranio-vertebral joints[127]

- Vertebral column malignancy or infection [124-126,128] which may preclude manual therapy

- A past history of cancer, particularly prostate, breast, lung, kidney.[124,125] The clinician should be aware of the possibility of bony metastases in these people

- Rheumatoid arthritis. Manipulation is precluded and also strong end of range techniques

- Long-term steroid use may have resulted in osteoporosis or soft tissue damage thus strong techniques are precluded

- Osteoporosis

- Systemically unwell generally, perhaps associated with significant weight loss for no apparent reason or fever [2,124,125]

- Structural deformity which has not been investigated or is recent in onset since the whiplash injury [124,125]

- Other conditions and syndromes associated with instability or hypermobility.

Evidence Summary 14   Level

Serious pathology (red flags)

- Symptoms needing urgent investigation: bilateral paraesthesia, gait disturbance, spastic paresis, positive Lhermittes sign, hyper reflexia, nerve root signs at more than two adjacent levels, progressively worsening neurological signs, symptoms of upper cervical instability, non-mechanical pain which is unremitting and severe   IV

- Symptoms that should be seen as precautions to treatment: positive stress tests of the cranio-vertebral joints, vertebral column malignancy or infection, a past history of cancer, rheumatoid arthritis, long-term steroid use, osteoporosis, systemically unwell generally, structural deformity, other conditions and syndromes associated with instability or hypermobility   IV

3.6.5 The physical examination

Physiotherapists should use findings from an assessment to develop hypotheses about people's condition and decide upon interventions that are likely to be effective, using their clinical reasoning skills. On subsequent visits people with WAD need to be reassessed to ensure that management and treatment plans can be altered as appropriate. The following is an outline of the physical examination and further details can be found in the recommended textbooks (section 15).

3.6.5.1 Observation

The following should be noted on observation:

- Posture

- Willingness to move head and neck

- Muscle bulk and tone

- Soft tissues

- Swelling

- Observed attitudes and feelings.

3.6.5.2 Movement

A comparative study (n=203) found that WAD reduced range of neck movement to the extent that people could correctly be categorised as either asymptomatic or having WAD on the basis of primary and conjunct range of movement, age and gender.[130] This emphasises the value of careful physical examination of movement at the assessment stage.

The physiotherapist should assess the following movements:

- Active movement of the cervical spine, thoracic spine and upper limbs
- Functional movements
- Quality of movement and range of movement
- The effect of movement on pain or other symptoms.

Physiotherapists may also assess:

- Passive physiological intervertebral movements (PPIVMs)
- Passive accessory intervertebral movements (PAIVMs)
- Combined and repeated movements with compression/over pressure
- Combined and repeated movements with and without compression or distraction.

3.6.5.3 Neurological tests

The integrity and mobility of the nervous system needs to be examined and tests should include:

- The integrity of the nervous system including testing myotomes, dermatomes and reflexes when indicated by the distribution of the symptoms
- Mobility tests may include passive neck flexion (PNF), upper limb tension tests (ULTT), passive knee bend, straight leg raise (SLR) and the slump test
- The plantar response should be examined to exclude an upper motor neurone lesion
- Tests for clonus, should be carried out to exclude an upper motor neurone lesion.

Response to the slump test in females (n=60) has been investigated. Those with neck pain following whiplash injury (n=20) were compared with asymptomatic women (n=40).[131] The group with neck pain were more limited in range of knee extension and experienced a significant increase in cervical symptoms suggesting that a pathological change of the neural system may contribute to neck pain.

3.6.5.4 Muscle tests

Muscle tests should include the assessment of muscle strength, control and length, and isometric contraction. Physiotherapists should be aware of a study comparing people with WAD with asymptomatic volunteers. People with WAD (n=12) were found to use superficial neck flexors more than asymptomatic volunteers (n=12). A possible explanation is that the use of superficial flexors was compensating for poor motor control in the deep neck flexor muscles.[132] This suggests that physiotherapy assessment for people with WAD should include assessment of dynamic control of posture and movement.

3.6.5.5 Proprioception

On assessment of proprioception people with WAD (n=11) demonstrated a deficit in their ability to reproduce a target position of the neck or to find a neutral position of the neck when compared with a control group of matched asymptomatic people (n=11). This suggests the importance of retraining proprioception after whiplash injury.[133]

3.6.5.6 Palpation

Palpation should include the cervical spine, thoracic spine and may include the head, face, upper limbs as appropriate. Note should be taken of the following:

- Skin temperature
- Localised increased skin moisture
- Presence of oedema or effusion
- Mobility and feel of superficial tissue

- Muscle spasm

- Tenderness

- Trigger points

- Bony prominence

- Factors that provoke or reduce pain.

Accessory movements may be included in the examination in order to identify and localise the symptomatic joint and adjacent joint motion.

3.6.5.7 Special tests

Special tests are recommended in specific circumstances as outlined below:

- **Vertebro basilar insufficiency.** Guidance has been produced in the UK as a joint venture between the Manipulation Association of Chartered Physiotherapists and the Society of Orthopaedic Medicine.[134] This intends to provide an evidence-based approach to vertebral artery insufficiency testing prior to cervical manipulation. The guidance highlights signs and symptoms that should be considered in the light of present research. It stresses that a recent or past history of whiplash is a risk factor in vascular accidents following cervical manipulation. Previous damage to the blood vessel wall may predispose the artery to further damage when cervical manipulation is applied.

- **Thoracic outlet syndrome.** Various tests for this complex syndrome have been described and include the Allen Test, Adson's manoeuvre and provocative elevation tests.[128]

- <u>Upper cervical stability.</u> Results from the Delphi survey indicated a high level of consensus that physiotherapists should test for instability in the presence of certain signs (inability to support the head, dysphagia, tongue paraesthesia, a metallic taste in the mouth, facial or lip paraesthesia, bilateral limb paraesthesia, quadrilateral limb paraesthesia, nystagmus, gait disturbance). **However the GDG was concerned that this response was misleading and agreed unanimously that extreme caution should be taken when considering the use of tests for instability. The presence of the listed symptoms would suggest a need for referral for urgent medical investigation.** <u>Joint integrity testing should only be conducted by a specially trained physiotherapist.</u>

3.6.5.8 Investigations

In the case of serious injury or suspected serious injury, people with WAD may need referral for investigations e.g. x-rays, CT or MRI scans. In this event, physiotherapists should take advice from experts in this field and imaging should be in accordance with guidelines produced by the Royal College of Radiologists [135] (Appendix H).

However, for WAD injuries of grade 0 – III (section 3.2) studies indicate that neither X-ray nor MRI scan is capable of detecting injury. A Japanese prospective study compared x-rays of people with acute whiplash injury (n=488) and asymptomatic volunteers (n=495). There was no significant difference between the two groups in:

- Frequencies of non-lordotic neck posture

- Local angular kyphosis.

There was no significant association found between:

- Clinical symptoms and cervical curvature. [136]

A prospective study compared the MRI scans of the cerebrum and cervical spine of people with whiplash (n=40) and asymptomatic volunteers (n=20). Scans were taken within two days of injury and six months later. No significant difference was found between the two groups in terms of brain and neck images.

The physical examination

- Recent or previous whiplash is a risk factor for vascular accidents when considering cervical manipulation or pre-manipulative testing   III

- For a minority (serious injury or suspected serious injury), the assessment process may involve referral for investigations e.g. X-rays, CT scans or MRI scans   III

- Physiotherapists should examine people with WAD through:

  · observation and palpation

  · testing of movement, neurological and muscular integrity

  · proprioceptive skills

  · relevant special tests   IV

- Expert opinion suggests that the presence of the following: inability to support head, dysphagia, tongue paraesthesia, a metallic taste in the mouth, facial or lip paraesthesia, bilateral limb paraesthesia, quadrilateral limb paraesthesia, nystagmus or gait disturbance suggests a need for further medical investigation rather than physiotherapeutic tests for instability. Joint integrity tests should only be applied by a physiotherapist with specialist training in this area   IV

3.6.6   Defining the aims of physiotherapy treatment

Clinical reasoning is a part of the assessment process and leads to the development of the aims of physiotherapy treatment. The Delphi questionnaire tackled this issue with a view to agreeing on some general aims of treatment. There was consensus that the aims of physiotherapy should be to relieve symptoms, improve function, facilitate empowerment and get the person back to normal activity/work.

Delphi findings indicate that the general aims of treatment for people with WAD are to:

- Improve function (*unanimity* 100%)

- Facilitate empowerment of the person with WAD (*unanimity* 100%)

- Get the person with WAD back to normal activity or work (*unanimity* 100%)

- Relieve symptoms (*consensus* 93%).

The general aims of treatment for people with WAD

- Improve function (*unanimity* 100%)   IV

- Facilitate empowerment of the person with WAD (*unanimity* 100%)   IV

- Get the person with WAD back to normal activity or work (*unanimity* 100%)   IV

- Relieve symptoms (*consensus* 93%)   IV

3.7   Pharmacological pain relief

There are no national guidelines on pharmacological pain relief for people with WAD.

A systematic review involving people with non-specific neck pain[138] found insufficient evidence when investigating the effectiveness of simple analgesia (paracetamol, opioids) or non-steroidal anti-inflammatory drugs (NSAIDs).

Evidence-based guidelines produced by PRODIGY[139] extrapolated information from research in other acute and chronic pain conditions. These recommend:

- Regular use of paracetamol in the first instance, particularly during the initial stage after injury when natural recovery is expected

- Progression to regular use of NSAIDs when paracetamol alone is inadequate and where there are no contraindications. NSAIDs are likely to offer short-term pain relief and there seems to be little difference between the different NSAIDs available.

There is, however, a difference in the risk of adverse events between different NSAIDs, with Ibuprofen having the lowest and azapropazone the highest risk. The newer cyclo-oxygenase 2 (Cox-2) inhibitors are associated with less gastrointestinal toxicity than older NSAIDs, however they may also be associated with more serious thrombotic cardiovascular events.[138] **Readers should note that some Cox-2 inhibitors have been taken off the market because of their side effects.** Those at risk of developing serious gastrointestinal adverse effects should also be given a gastroprotective agent with an NSAID. The PRODIGY guidelines [139] should be referred to for an indication of those at risk and which gastroprotective agents are suitable. A combination of paracetamol and codeine may be needed if paracetamol or NSAIDs do not give adequate pain relief on their own. Separate prescriptions of the two drugs are preferred to help find the safest and most effective dose to match the person's requirements.

Physiotherapists must be aware of their own personal scope of practice and limit their advice and treatment to areas in which they can demonstrate their ability to work safely and competently.[157]

Evidence Summary 17   Level

Advising on pain relief for people with WAD

- Paracetamol is likely to be the best painkiller immediately after injury

- NSAIDs should be used if paracetamol is ineffective

- Combined paracetamol and codeine may be necessary where a person experiences a great deal of pain

- Possible side effects of drugs should always be considered

- Physiotherapists must advise within the scope of their practice.   IV

Recommendations for the physiotherapy assessment and examination of people with WAD

Grade

Valid consent (ES 10)

Valid consent should be sought and recorded in line with national standards and guidance, and local organisational policy   C

Access to physiotherapy service (ES11, 12)

Physiotherapists should prioritise entry into the physiotherapy service by:

- Screening individual people   C

- Providing a physiotherapy service in an accident and emergency department   C

- Assessing individual people by telephone   C

Physiotherapists should prioritise people who:

- Find their activities of daily living disrupted as a result of WAD   C

- Are unable to work as a result of WAD   C

- Have a more recent injury   C

Subjective assessment (ES 13)

A thorough subjective assessment is essential to help plan subsequent examination and treatment.   Good practice point

Serious pathology (red flags) (ES 14)

- People with WAD must be screened for red flags

  Good practice point

- People with bilateral paraesthesia, gait disturbance, spastic paresis, positive Lhermittes sign, hyper reflexia, nerve root signs at more than two adjacent levels, progressively worsening neurological signs, symptoms of upper cervical instability, non-mechanical pain which is unremitting and severe must be referred immediately to the nearest accident and emergency department

  Good practice point

- People with positive stress tests of the cranio-vertebral joints, vertebral column malignancy or infection, a past history of cancer, rheumatoid arthritis, long-term steroid use, osteoporosis, systemically unwell generally, structural deformity, other conditions and syndromes associated with instability or hypermobility should be treated with caution

  Good practice point

The physical examination (ES 15)

- Joint instability testing should only be conducted by a specially trained physiotherapist

  Good practice point

- Cervical manipulation and pre-manipulative testing techniques should be avoided for people with WAD

  Good practice point

- Physiotherapists need to know when special tests and investigations are indicated and how to carry out the tests or refer people appropriately

  Good practice point

- **People with WAD presenting with signs and symptoms of instability must immediately be referred for further investigation**

  Good practice point

- Inexperienced physiotherapists must know when to ask advice from senior staff

  Good practice point

Defining the aims of physiotherapy treatment (ES 16)

Although treatment is tailored to individual needs, general aims of physiotherapy treatment should be to:

- Improve function   C
- Facilitate empowerment of the person with WAD   C
- Return the person to normal activity/work   C
- Relieve symptoms   C

Advising on pain relief (ES 17)

- Physiotherapists should refer to local guidelines for prescription of analgesia. Good practice point

- Where guidelines do not exist physiotherapists and people with WAD should seek appropriate medical advice.

  Good practice point

Physiotherapy interventions

This section considers which physiotherapy interventions are most effective in assisting people with WAD to return to normal activity and how and when physiotherapists should treat people with WAD. The evidence and recommendations in this section are based on a systematic review of the research as has been described earlier in sections 2.3. and 2.4. The evidence from individual randomised controlled trials (RCTs) of people with whiplash injuries was reviewed. For areas where no whiplash studies were available, systematic reviews and more recent RCTs of people with mechanical neck pain were included. The Delphi questionnaire was used where research evidence was incomplete. This section is broken into three discrete sections:

- Acute WAD (the first two weeks after whiplash injury)
- Subacute WAD (after two weeks and up to12 weeks after whiplash injury)
- Chronic WAD (more than 12 weeks after whiplash injury).

This reflects the way in which the research evidence is presented in the literature.

Recommendations are made on the basis of the systematic review of the literature where evidence exists. Little high quality research is available on the physiotherapy treatment for people with WAD. As a result much of the evidence and some of the recommendations are addressed by considering the evidence in non-specific chronic neck pain and by using the results of the Delphi questionnaire.

4.1 Acute WAD (zero to two weeks after whiplash injury)

4.1.1 The effect of soft collars

One quasi-randomised clinical controlled trial (n=196) compared a soft collar worn as much as possible for the first two weeks after a whiplash injury with a control group. Both groups were advised to rest and take analgesia (NSAIDs) at the discretion of the treating physician and followed up after six weeks.[36] The methodological quality of this study was poor (PEDro 3/10); people were not assigned randomly to groups, their medical record numbers were used by allocating odd numbers to the collar group and even numbers to the control group. Outcome measurement was not blinded. Of those originally allocated to the groups,[54] (22%) did not attend the follow up at six weeks and were not included in the analysis, suggesting that an intention-to-treat analysis was not used. The length of follow up was only six weeks, which is not long enough to give any indication of the long-term effects of using a cervical collar. The difference between the groups was not statistically significant for global perceived pain, with 85% of the collar and 80% of the control groups reporting a reduction in pain or no pain after six weeks, and 5% and 8% of the collar and control groups, respectively reporting worse pain.

In view of the poor quality of the evidence, a question about the use of soft collars was included in the Delphi questionnaire. Delphi findings indicate that soft collars should not be used to enhance the effect of rest and analgesia in reducing pain (*majority view* 74%)

Evidence Summary 18	Level
Soft collars	
• Combining a soft collar, rest and analgesia is equally effective as rest and analgesia (downgraded for poor quality)	IIb
• Soft collars should not be used to enhance the effect of rest and analgesia in reducing pain (*majority view* 74%)	IV

4.1.2 The effect of other interventions to enhance the effect of rest and analgesia in reducing pain

Delphi findings indicate that, in the acute stage, the following techniques should be used to enhance the effect of rest and analgiesia in reducing pain:

- Active exercise (*unanimity* 100%)
- Advice about coping strategies (*unanimity* 100%)
- Education about the origin of pain (*consensus* 96%)
- An active exercise programme devised for each individual following assessment (*consensus* 93%)
- A general active exercise programme devised for people with WAD (*consensus* 92%)
- Soft tissue techniques (*majority view* 59%)
- TENS (*majority view* 52%)
- Relaxation (*majority view* 52%).

Delphi findings indicate that, in the acute stage, the following techniques should not be used to enhance the effect of rest and analgesia in reducing pain:

- Infrared light (*consensus* 85%)
- Traction (*consensus* 76%)
- Laser treatment (*majority view* 65%)
- Interferential therapy (*majority view* 63%)
- Ultrasound treatment (*majority view* 63%).

The Delphi findings neither support nor refute the use of manual mobilisation, massage or acupuncture.

In the absence of any research evidence, the evidence for and against interventions designed to enhance the effect of rest and analgesia in reducing pain is based on level IV Delphi findings.

Evidence Summary 19

Other interventions to enhance the effect of rest and analgesia in reducing pain

Interventions that enhance the effect of rest and analgesia in reducing pain:

	Level
• Active exercise (*unanimity* 100%)	IV
• Advice about coping strategies (*unanimity* 100%)	IV
• Education about the origin of pain (*consensus* 96%)	IV
• An active exercise programme devised for each individual following assessment (*consensus* 93%)	IV
• A general active exercise programme devised for people with WAD (*consensus* 92%)	IV
• Soft tissue techniques (*majority view* 59%)	IV
• TENS (*majority view* 52%)	IV
• Relaxation (*majority view* 52%)	IV

Interventions that **do not** enhance the effect of rest and analgesia in reducing pain:

• Infrared light (*consensus* 85%)	IV
• Traction (*consensus* 76%)	IV
• Laser treatment (*majority view* 65%)	IV
• Interferential therapy (*majority view* 63%)	IV
• Ultrasound treatment (*majority view* 63%)	IV

There was no consensus about the use of manual mobilisation, massage or acupuncture.

4.1.3 Early activity versus initial rest and soft collar

One RCT of people who had sustained a whiplash injury (n=178) compared return to normal activities ('act as usual') without sick leave or use of a collar with 14 days sick leave and use of a soft cervical collar.[33] This was a well-conducted RCT (PEDro 6/10), which had blind outcome assessment, but did not use intention-to-treat analysis. A visual analogue scale (VAS) was used to measure neck pain and headache before and at follow up. However no details of this measure were given. The overall improvement in neck pain VAS over six months was similar in the two groups, although the rest group improved more in the first six weeks than the 'act as usual' group, which improved more after the six-week follow up. There were no differences between the groups in relation to neck and shoulder movement immediately after treatment or at the six-month follow up. The person's global perceived improvement was also similar after six months, with 21% of the 'act as usual' and 22% of the rest group reporting more symptoms, and less symptoms reported by 66% and 63% of the 'act as usual' and rest groups, respectively.

Evidence Summary 20   Level

Returning to normal activity

- Returning to normal activities is as beneficial as rest and use of a neck collar in the first 2 weeks after a whiplash injury   Ib

4.1.4 Early manual mobilisation techniques versus initial rest and soft collar

Two RCTs compared the use of manual mobilisation techniques and exercise with rest in a soft collar for the first two or three weeks after injury.[32,40]

In the RCT by Bonk et al, manual mobilisation was given three times in the first week and twice in each of the second and third weeks after injury.[32] Unspecified exercises to increase mobility were carried out at each session by the person, as well as strengthening and isometric exercises. In the third week the active group was given interscapular muscle strengthening exercises and postural advice. All subjects (n=97) were followed up at one, two, three, six and 12 weeks. The methodological quality was good (PEDro 5/10). However, this RCT has serious flaws that may have biased the results, as outcome assessment was not blinded and no intention-to-treat analysis was used. All six of those who withdrew from the study were in the active group; one experienced neurological signs and the other five were removed because they were non-compliant with therapy, and these five have not been included in the analysis of the results. Neck pain in the active group improved much quicker than in the rest group; the difference in prevalence of neck pain in the two groups was statistically significant after six weeks (11% versus 62%, respectively). However by the 12 week follow up there was little difference in neck pain reported (2% versus 16%, respectively). No statistically significant differences were reported between the active and rest groups in relation to range of movement at six or 12 weeks.

In the other RCT[40], people in the active group were given unspecified home exercises every hour, within the limits of pain, between manual mobilisation sessions with the therapist. Manual mobilisation (Maitland) of repetitive and passive movements was carried out within the person's tolerance. A blind assessor measured outcomes (n=61) after 4 and 8 weeks. This RCT was given a high score for methodological quality (PEDro 6/10). However, the trial is small and as no intention-to-treat analysis was used, the exclusion of ten people (five from each group) from the analysis due to incomplete data reduces the size and power of the study even further. Initial scores for pain and range of movement were different in the two groups. Statistically significant improvements from baseline were seen in pain scores in both groups at four weeks and in the active treatment group at eight weeks. There were also statistically significant improvements seen in cervical movement at four weeks in the active group and in both groups after eight weeks. Pain scores were significantly lower at four weeks in the active treatment group than in the rest group, and both pain scores and cervical movement had improved significantly more at eight weeks in the group receiving active therapy than in the rest group.

No evidence regarding the long-term benefit of early mobilisation for whiplash injuries is available; the follow up period of these studies was 8–12 weeks.

In view of the quality issues of these studies, a question was included in the Delphi process. Delphi findings indicate that, in the acute stage, early manual mobilisation is:

- More effective than rest and a soft collar in improving neck range of movement (*consensus* 81%)

- More effective than initial rest in improving function (*consensus* 81%).

Thus, in addition to the level **IIa** evidence, there is some level **IV** evidence that manual mobilisation may be more effective than initial rest and a soft collar in the acute stage.

Evidence Summary 21	Level
Manual mobilisation versus initial rest and a soft collar	

- Early manual mobilisation reduces levels of pain more than initial rest IIa (down-graded for poor quality)

- Early manual mobilisation is more effective than rest and a soft collar in improving neck range of movement (*consensus* 81%) · IV

- Early manual mobilisation is more effective than initial rest in improving function (*consensus* 81%) · IV

4.1.5 Early exercise and advice versus initial rest and soft collar

The two RCTs by Bonk et al[32] and Mealy et al[40] reviewed in the previous section show that unspecified exercises carried out with manual mobilisation by a therapist are more effective for reducing pain than rest in the initial 2 weeks after a whiplash injury.

Another RCT (n=97) by Rosenfeld et al,[43] compared a McKenzie active exercise and posture protocol with a standard leaflet containing information on the injury and advice on posture and suitable activities. The early exercise group were instructed in performing hourly home exercises consisting of gentle, active, rotational movements of small-range and amplitude, ten times in both directions. The standard leaflet contained advice to rest and wear a soft collar for a few weeks before beginning active movement. The study compared the effects of starting these treatment protocols within 96 hours of the injury with waiting until 14 days after the injury to begin the treatments. During the wait the two delayed treatment groups were not prescribed any therapy, apart from any instructions they had received from the referring physician. Including these two extra groups in the study design meant that the group sizes were small (ranging from 21 to 23 people in each group).

The final update search revealed another paper by Rosenfeld et al[29] giving 3-year follow-up data for this RCT. The methods and results were reported more thoroughly in the follow-up paper than they had been in the original. With the details from the updated paper the methodological quality was classified as high (PEDro 7/10). Use of intention-to-treat was discussed; when a worst-case scenario was used no differences were seen between those on active and standard treatments. Without an intention-to-treat analysis the results of the study show a statistically significant greater reduction in pain for the two groups receiving the active exercise therapy than the groups who had the standard treatment (p<0.001). No differences were seen however in the mean change in range of movement between the two treatment protocols. Low pain scores of less than 10mm on a 100mm visual analogue scale were reported by 52% (11/21) of the early active exercise group and 30% (7/23) of the early standard therapy group, which is not a statistically significant difference. There was a combined effect of treatment and time factor on the reduction of pain (p=0.04) and improvement of cervical flexion (p=0.01). Active exercise was more effective when administered within 96 hours of the accident and standard therapy achieved better results when delayed for 2 weeks. After three years the difference between the active and the standard treatment in the change in pain intensity was still statistically significant. However, the combined effect of intervention and timing was not statistically significant at the three-year follow-up.

Early exercise and advice versus initial rest and soft collar

- There is greater reduction of pain at 6 months after early active exercise and postural advice consistent with McKenzie principles than an early standard advice leaflet   Ib

- There is no difference in range of movement after early active exercise and early standard advice given within 96 hours of a whiplash injury   Ib

- Active exercise has the greatest effect on pain reduction if administered within 96 hours of a whiplash injury occurring   Ib

4.1.6 Early physiotherapy programme versus initial rest and soft collar

One quasi-randomised study by Pennie & Agambar[41] (n=135) allocated participants to either a standard treatment of two weeks rest in a neck collar (either soft collar or moulded thermoplastic polyethylene foam) and a taught unspecified programme of active neck exercises, or physiotherapy (traction and advice on posture and home exercises). The methodological quality of this study was poor (PEDro 3/10). It is impossible to tell from the report of this study if true randomisation took place or not. Random allocation has been made on the basis of the casualty number without any further detail given. Other serious flaws include gender and social class differences in the two groups, outcome assessment was not blind and no intention-to-treat analysis was used. The number of non-attendees was similar in both groups, with 13 from each group missing at their 6-8 week follow up, and four and three people missing from the collar and physiotherapy groups respectively, for the five months follow up. There was no statistically significant difference between the two groups in relation to reduction in neck pain, total movement or people's subjective assessment, with 98% (64/70) in the collar group and 97% (56/58) in the physiotherapy group reporting 'cured' or 'improved' symptoms 5 months after their accidents.

In view of the poor quality of the study, a question was included in the Delphi process. Delphi findings indicate that, in the first two weeks after injury:

- Early physiotherapy 'as usual' is more effective than initial rest followed by an exercise routine in improving function (*majority view* 52%)

Thus there is some level **IV** evidence that an early physiotherapy programme may be more effective than initial rest and a soft collar in the acute stage.

Early physiotherapy programme versus initial rest and soft collar

- Early physiotherapy 'as usual' is more effective than initial rest followed by an exercise routine in improving function (*majority view* 52%)   IV

4.1.7 Early education and advice versus initial rest & other modalities

One RCT reported in two papers by McKinney et al[38,39] was a single-blind RCT that compared a tailored programme of outpatient physiotherapy, with advice on self-management, with a group advised to rest for two weeks before starting activities. Physiotherapy was devised, after the person was assessed, from resources available at the hospital, typically the programme included active exercises and manual mobilisation (McKenzie & Maitland principles), hot and cold applications, short-wave diathermy, hydrotherapy and traction. The advice group were also assessed by the physiotherapist and given advice on posture, unspecified active exercises (demonstrated), and appropriate use of painkillers, collars, heat sources and muscle relaxation. Everyone was seen within 48 hours of the accident and fitted with a soft foam collar and given analgesia (co-dydramol 1000mg 6-hourly). Enrolment to the rest group was stopped early, as the outcomes measured after two months in this group were significantly poorer than those in the other two groups, and it was felt that it was unethical to withhold instruction on effective mobilisation to this group of people. The methodological quality of this RCT was high (PEDro 6/10). No intention-to-treat analysis was used, however. 77 (31%) of the original sample (n=247) did not attend the two-month follow up and 80 (32%) were not available for the two-year follow up. The non-attendees were distributed evenly between the three groups and did not differ significantly in age, sex or initial severity from those who attended the follow up. After two months there were no statistically significant differences between the physiotherapy and advice groups in either pain or range of movement. However, at the 2 year follow up 44% (24/54) of the physiotherapy group and 46% (12/26) of the rest group still had symptoms, whereas only 23% (11/48) of the advice group had persistent symptoms; this was a statistically significant difference.

Evidence Summary 24   Level

Early education and advice versus initial rest and other modalities

- Early physiotherapy advice on self-management is more effective in reducing persistent self-reported symptoms in the long term than an early programme of tailored physiotherapy   Ib

- Early physiotherapy advice on self-management was equally as effective as a tailored physiotherapy programme in the short term   Ib

4.1.8 Early electrotherapy versus use of neck collar

One RCT (n=40) by Foley-Nolan et al compared active pulsed electromagnetic therapy (PEMT) units with dummy units within 72 hours of an accident.[35] Both the active and the dummy units were embedded in a collar. Participants were advised to wear the neck collars for 8 hours a day throughout the 12 week study period and to mobilise their necks hourly within pain-free range. NSAIDS were also prescribed and amount used recorded. After four weeks, nine study participants (45%) in the active and 12 (60%) in the dummy group were unhappy with their progress and were referred to a physiotherapist for individualised therapy twice a week for six weeks (typically included hot packs, pulsed wave diathermy, ultrasound & active repetitive movements). The results for these people were analysed according to an intention-to-treat analysis, i.e. in the group to which they had been randomly assigned. This may have affected the overall results as a large proportion of both groups received similar treatment programmes after four weeks in the study. The RCT achieved a high score for methodological quality (PEDro 9/10). The active group improved in terms of pain (after two weeks and four weeks) and this was statistically significant but it was not maintained (after 12 weeks). Significantly more people in the active PEMT group perceived their improvement as 'moderately' or 'much better' than those in the dummy group
at four weeks (85% (17/20) vs. 35% (7/20), respectively; p=0.001). The difference was less after 12 weeks, 85% for the active PEMT group compared with 60% for the control group.

Evidence Summary 25   Level

Early electrotherapy versus use of neck collar

- Early PEMT administered in a neck collar reduced pain faster than a neck collar with no PEMT, but there was no difference in pain reduction at 12 weeks   Ib

- Perceived improvement was greater in the PEMT collar group than the collar with no PEMT group   Ib

In this clinical trial, specially made cervical collars containing PEMT units were worn for eight hours a day throughout the 12 weeks of the study. This is very different from the exposure to PEMT a person with WAD would normally have in a physiotherapy department in the UK. Despite the fact that the evidence supporting the use of PEMT was the result of a well-conducted RCT, the GDG did not consider the results are generalisable to people with WAD who receive conventional PEMT in the UK today. Therefore, after much discussion the GDG has decided that this evidence cannot be used as the basis of a recommendation on the effectiveness of the conventional use of PEMT.

Soft collars

- The use of soft collars is not recommended (ES 18)   C

Manual mobilisation

- Manual mobilisation shoud be considered for the reduction of neck pain in the
  initial stages (ES 21)   B

- Manual mobilisation should be considered to increase neck range
  of movement (ES 21)   C

- Manual mobilisation should be considered to improve function (ES 21)   C

- Soft tissue techniques should be considered for the reduction of pain (ES 19)   C

Exercise therapy

- Active exercise should be used to reduce pain (ES 19 and 22)   A

- Active exercise for pain reduction should be started within four days of injury (ES 22)   A

- An active exercise programme devised for each individual following assessment should be
  considered for the reduction of pain (ES 19)   C

Education and advice

- Advice on self-management should be provided, to reduce patients' symptoms (ES 24)   A

- Returning to normal activities as soon as possible should be encouraged (ES 20)   A

- Providing education about the origin of the pain should be considered for reducing
  pain (ES 19)   C

- Providing advice about coping strategies may be helpful for the reduction of pain (ES 19)   C

- Relaxation should be considered for reducing pain (ES 19)   C

Physical agents (including electrotherapy)

- The use of TENS should be considered for reducing pain (ES 19)   C

- The following are unlikely to be effective in reducing pain: (ES 19)   C
    Traction
    Infrared light
    Interferential therapy
    Ultrasound treatment
    Laser treatment

- There is insufficient evidence to support or refute the use of the following: (ES 19)
    Massage   C
    Acupuncture   C
    PEMT   Good practice point

4.2.1 Manipulation and manual mobilisation

There were no studies found exploring the effects of manipulation in people with only whiplash injuries. However there was a systematic review of the literature, from 1966 to January 1998, on the effectiveness of manipulation and manual mobilisation in acute and chronic mechanical neck disorders including whiplash injuries.[140] The review made the following conclusions from the RCTs and quasi-RCTs found:

- No benefit was found in using manipulation alone in a single session to decrease pain [two large RCTs], and there was insufficient evidence on the effectiveness of more than one session in reducing pain [four small RCTs]

- No difference was found in pain and function when manual mobilisation alone was compared with a control group [one small RCT], other modalities (ice, TENS) [one small RCT], acupuncture [one small RCT] or a single manipulation [two small RCTs].

- A combination of manipulation and manual mobilisation showed no more benefit in decreased pain than a control group, and there was insufficient evidence on the effectiveness of combined manipulation and manual mobilisation to improve function [one small RCT].

Another systematic review of the evidence on neck pain found two trials on manipulation of reasonable quality with positive outcomes.[141] The review also found two trials that did not obtain high methodological quality scores, one with positive outcomes and the other with equivocal or negative outcomes for manipulation. Three manual mobilisation trials were found, all of which were lower methodological quality and further details were not reported. There was insufficient detail on specific interventions used to draw conclusions on the effectiveness of manipulation or manual mobilisation from this review.

However, Delphi findings indicate that, in the subacute stage:

- Combined manipulation and manual mobilisation reduces pain (*majority view* 52%)

- Combined manipulation and manual mobilisation improves function (*majority view* 52%)

- Manipulation alone does not reduce pain (*majority view* 55%).

Delphi findings are inconclusive on the following, that in the subacute stage:

- Manual mobilisation alone reduces pain

- Manual mobilisation is more effective than a combination of ice and TENS in reducing pain

- Manual mobilisation is more effective than acupuncture in reducing pain

- Manual mobilisation is more effective than a single manipulation in reducing pain.

Thus there is some level **IV** evidence that manual therapy may be of benefit at the subacute stage.

Evidence Summary 26	Level
Manual therapy	
• Combined manipulation and manual mobilisation may reduce pain (*majority view* 52%)	IV
• Combined manipulation and manual mobilisation may improve function (*majority view* 52%)	IV

4.2.2 Adverse events from cervical manipulation

There is some indication of the incidence of adverse events for people with mechanical neck pain. One systematic review found the risk of adverse events from cervical manipulation difficult to estimate accurately due to the poor quality of the literature.[140] However, the review suggests the estimate of serious adverse events ranges from one in 20,000 to 5–10 in 10 million cervical manipulations. The risk of minor or moderate events, such as headache or nausea, was said to range from one in 3,020 to one in 7,550 cervical manipulations. In one of the studies risk of stroke from cervical manipulation (0.001%) was compared with the risk of death from gastrointestinal bleeding following use of NSAIDS (less than or equal to 0.04%).[142]

A more recent systematic review of prospective studies by Stevinson and Ernst estimated that minor, transient adverse effects occur in approximately half of all people receiving spinal manipulation.[143] The most common serious adverse events from cervical spinal manipulation were vertebrobasilar accidents, particularly for those under 45 years of age. The most reliable estimate given was that 'for every 100,000 people under 45 years receiving chiropractic treatment, approximately 1.3 cases of vertebrobasilar accidents attributable to that treatment would be observed within 1 week of manipulation'.

Results of the Delphi survey indicated a high level of consensus that, in the subacute stage, the risk of serious adverse events (eg vertebrobasilar accidents) from manipulation is low. **However the GDG urges caution because whiplash has been identified as a risk factor in vascular accidents following cervical manipulation[134] (section 3.6.5.7 and evidence summary 15).**

Delphi findings indicate that, in the subacute stage:

* The risk of serious adverse events (eg vertebrobasilar accidents) from manipulation is low (*consensus* 93%)

* There is no agreement on whether minor or moderate adverse events (eg headache or nausea) occur in around half of all people receiving cervical manipulation.

Evidence Summary 27   Level

Adverse effects from cervical manipulation

* For mechanical neck pain, the risk of serious adverse events from cervical manipulation is low   III

* A history of whiplash injury is a risk factor for vascular accidents following cervical manipulation   IV

4.2.3 Exercise therapy

One RCT by Soderlund et al (n=53)[44] compared regular treatment, consisting of three specified exercises three times a day to restore movement with the same regular treatment, plus another exercise to improve 'kinaesthetic sensibility and coordination'. All participants also received advice on posture and staying active. The methodological quality of this RCT was low (PEDro 4/10), as outcome assessment was not blinded and no intention-to-treat analysis was used. A total of 13 people (20%) dropped out, roughly the same number from each group before the end of the study. There was also poor adherence to the exercises, with only 41% of all people completing the exercises for more than 5 days a week. The trial found only a small difference in improvement in pain level and range of movement in the group receiving the additional exercise compared with the regular exercise group, which was not statistically significant.

A systematic review[144] of the evidence on exercise in mechanical neck disorders described the same RCT for whiplash, and included another that is reviewed later in the section on chronic whiplash. The other RCTs found in this review included people with chronic or recurrent neck pain and are also reviewed in a later section.

Evidence Summary 28   Level

Exercise therapy

* There appears to be no additional benefit from including kinaesthetic exercise to a programme of functional improvement exercises. (down-graded for poor quality)   IIa

4.2.4 Multimodal/multidisciplinary packages and psychosocial approaches

An RCT by Provinciali et al compared the effect of a multimodal treatment (postural training, manual techniques and psychological support) with a treatment programme of physical agents alone (including TENS, PEMT and ultrasound).[42] This RCT included 60 people within 60 days of a whiplash injury. The methodological quality was good (PEDro 6/10). Outcome assessment was blind and nobody was lost to follow up. After adjusting for baseline differences, the pain intensity was significantly less for those in the multimodal group than those given physical agents (1.9 vs. 4.8 on a 10-point visual analogue scale, p<0.0001). People's subjective assessment of the effectiveness of treatment they received was also significantly different in the two groups (2 for multimodal group vs. −1 in the physical agents group, on a scale from 3 [total recovery] to −3 [complete disability]). The average delay in returning to work was significantly less for the multimodal group than the physical agents group (38.4 days, SD 10.5 vs. 54.3 days, SD 18.4).

A systematic overview of the evidence found one systematic review and two more recent RCTs in people with chronic neck pain, which have been included in a later section, but none were found in people with sub acute neck pain.[14]

One systematic review of multidisciplinary biopsychosocial rehabilitation in people with subacute low back pain, from which it may be possible to extrapolate to cervical neck pain was found.[145] The only two relevant studies, both of low methodological quality, provide moderate evidence to show that multidisciplinary rehabilitation, which includes an occupational health element, helps get people back to work faster, reduces sick leave and lessens subjective functional impairment.

Evidence Summary 29   Level

Multimodal/multidisciplinary packages and psychosocial approaches

- A multimodal programme (including postural training, manual technique and psychological support) is more effective for whiplash injuries than a programme of physical agents, as rated by participants. The programme reduces pain and speeds their return to work   Ia

4.2.5 Acupuncture

No studies were found on the effects of acupuncture for people with acute whiplash. However one systematic review of acute and chronic non-specific neck pain investigated the effects of acupuncture.[146] The review found eight studies of reasonable quality comparing acupuncture with a range of therapies and controls. Five of these studies gave negative results for acupuncture and only three achieved positive results. However results were conflicting and acupuncture was not superior to any one modality in any of the trials. The authors concluded that the evidence did not support the use of acupuncture in the treatment of neck pain.

Delphi findings indicate that, in the subacute stage, acupuncture is effective in reducing neck pain (*majority view* 52%)

Evidence Summary 30   level

Acupuncture

- Acupuncture may be effective in reducing neck pain (*majority view* 52%)   IV

- For non-specific neck pain, there was conflicting evidence about whether acupuncture was effective in reducing neck pain   Ia

4.2.6 Education and/or advice

No RCTs were found, other than the trial by McKinney looking at early advice which has previously been described, on the effects of education and advice on whiplash injuries.[38,39] Advice has been included in many of the RCTs but none study the effect of advice or education in isolation.

A Cochrane systematic review of people with non-specific neck pain identified three RCTs of patient education interventions. This review has been withdrawn from the Cochrane Library due to lack of recent updates.[147] They found too few studies using any one educational intervention to make any conclusive statement on the benefits or risks of patient education.

Delphi findings indicate that, in the subacute stage:

- Education is effective in improving neck function (*consensus* 96%)

- Advice about coping strategies is effective in enabling people to return to normal activities (*consensus* 96%).

Evidence Summary 31	Level
Education and/or advice	
• Education is effective in improving neck function (*consensus* 96%)	**IV**
• Advice about coping is effective in enabling people to return to normal activities (*consensus 96%*)	**IV**

4.2.7 Traction

No studies that specifically investigated the use of traction on people with whiplash were identified. However one systematic review of people with non-specific neck pain found three RCTs of poor quality studying traction versus various interventions, including heat, mobilisation, exercise, analgesics, neck collar, and no treatment.[148] Only one of the RCTs showed a positive result for traction. However, the review could not draw any conclusions from the RCTs included because the traction used was not standard across the studies and different additional therapies were used. Another systematic review (also withdrawn from the Cochrane Library due to lack of recent updates) found three RCTs that suggested that traction was ineffective, however there was insufficient power in the trials to make any conclusive judgements.[149]

Delphi findings indicate that, in the subacute stage, traction is **not effective** in reducing neck pain (*majority view* 52%)

Evidence Summary 32	Level
Traction	
• Traction is not effective in reducing neck pain (*majority view* 52%)	**IV**

4.2.8 Physical agents (including electrotherapy) and other interventions

A package of physical agents (TENS, PEMT and ultrasound) was compared with a multimodal treatment (postural training, manual techniques and psychological support) in an RCT described previously.[42] The results of this RCT suggest that physical agents are not as effective as a multimodal approach in reducing pain and speeding return to work. People who received the multimodal programme also assessed the effectiveness of the intervention higher than those receiving the package of physical agents.

A systematic review of rehabilitation interventions[150] found one RCT comparing TENS with use of a neck collar. It found no statistically significant difference in patient-assessed pain after a week or three months.

A Cochrane systematic review (withdrawn from Cochrane Library due to lack of recent updates) of physical modalities in people with mechanical neck disorders was found[149] The review had the following findings:

TENS: One RCT found no difference between TENS and a control treatment of collar, rest, education and analgesia.

Infrared light: One placebo-controlled trial found a statistically non-significant treatment effect for the use of infrared light, but there was insufficient power to draw a definite conclusion from this trial.

Laser: Three RCTs of laser therapy, when combined indicated that laser did not significantly reduce pain levels compared to the control treatment. However, there is insufficient power to make a conclusive statement about the ineffectiveness of laser therapy.

Delphi findings indicate that, in the subacute stage:

- Soft tissue techniques are effective in reducing neck pain (*consensus* 78%)

- Muscle retraining to include deep neck flexor activity is effective in improving function (*consensus* 78%)

- Massage is effective in reducing neck pain (*majority view* 65%)

- TENS is effective in reducing neck pain (*majority view* 59%).

Delphi findings indicate that, in the subacute stage, the following are not effective in reducing neck pain:

- Infrared light (*majority view* 63%)

- Interferential therapy (*majority view* 59%)

- Laser treatment (*majority view* 55%)

- Ultrasound treatment (*majority view* 52%)

Delphi findings are inconclusive on the benefits of phasic exercise in improving function and the benefits of using soft collars.

Evidence Summary 33	Level

Physical agents

• A package of physical agents was not as effective at reducing pain and reducing delays in returning to work as a multimodal programme	Ib
• Soft tissue techniques may be effective in reducing neck pain (*consensus* 78%)	IV
• Muscle retraining including deep neck flexor activity may be effective in improving function (*consensus* 78%)	IV
• Massage and TENS may be effective in reducing neck pain:	
· massage (*majority view* 65%)	IV
· TENS (*majority view* 59%)	IV
• The following physical agents are **unlikely to be effective** in reducing neck pain:	
· infrared light (*majority view* 63%)	IV
· interferential therapy (*majority view* 59%)	IV
· laser treatment (*majority view* 55%)	IV
· ultrasound (*majority view* 52%)	IV

For mechanical neck disorders:

• No difference was found between TENS and treatment with collar, rest, education and analgesia	Ia
• Infrared light and laser treatment were both ineffective compared to placebo or control therapy, but there was insufficient power to make any definite conclusions	Ia

Manipulation and manual mobilisation

- Combined manipulation and manual mobilisation should be considered for reducing pain (ES 26)   C

- Combined manipulation and manual mobilisation should be considered for improving function (ES 26)   C

- The risk of serious adverse events from cervical manipulation may be increased after whiplash injury (ES 27)   Good practice point

Exercise therapy

- There is unlikely to be any benefit in including kinaesthetic exercise in a programme of functional improvement exercise (ES 28)   B

- Muscle retraining including deep neck flexor activity may be effective in improving function (ES 33)   C

Multimodal packages

- A multimodal programme (including postural training, manual techniques and psychological support) should be used to reduce pain and speed return to work (ES 29)   A

Acupuncture

- The use of acupuncture cannot be supported or refuted (ES 30)   C

Education and advice

- Education should be considered for the improvement of neck function (ES 31)   C

- Advice about coping strategies should be considered, to enable people to return to normal activities (ES 31)   C

Physical agents (including electrotherapy)

The following treatments could be considered for the reduction of pain: (ES 33)   C

- TENS

- Massage

- Soft tissue techniques

The following treatments are unlikely to reduce neck pain: C

- Traction (ES 32)

- Infrared light (ES 33)

- Interferential therapy (ES 33)

- Laser treatment (ES 33)

- Ultrasound (ES 33)

4.3 Chronic WAD (more than 12 weeks after whiplash injury)

4.3.1 Manipulation and manual mobilisation

There were no studies found which considered the effects of manipulation in people with chronic whiplash injuries. However, one systematic review, included previously for sub acute WAD on the effectiveness of manipulation and manual mobilisation in acute and chronic mechanical neck disorders, was relevant.[140] The review drew the following conclusions from the RCTs and quasi-RCTs found:

- A single session of manipulation was not shown to decrease pain (2 large RCTs), and there was insufficient evidence regarding the effectiveness of more than one session of manipulation in reducing pain (4 small RCTs)

- No difference in functional improvement was found between the use of manipulation, high-technology exercise or combined low-technology exercise with manipulation. High-technology exercise and combined low-technology exercise with manipulation tended to improve long-term pain levels most. Patient satisfaction improved more with combined low-technology exercise with manipulation [one large RCT]. In these studies high-technology exercise made use of a machine that allowed isolated testing and exercise of the cervical extensors and rotators and low-technology exercise comprised cervical strengthening exercises using a simple pulley system for weight resistance.[151]

- No difference was found in pain and function when manual mobilisation alone was compared with a control group [one small RCT], other modalities (ice, TENS) [one small RCT], acupuncture [one small RCT] or a single manipulation [two small RCTs]

- A combination of manipulation and manual mobilisation showed no more benefit in decreasing pain than a control group, and there was insufficient evidence on the effectiveness of combined manipulation and manual mobilisation in improving function [one small RCT].

Two-year follow-up data[27] was found in the update search for one of the RCTs in the systematic review.[151] The conclusions did not change from the previous report, with people in both exercise groups reporting lower pain levels than the group that received spinal manipulation alone.

Another review of the literature[152] on manipulation and mobilisation for treating chronic pain found the same RCTs as Gross et al.[140] The authors of this review concluded that manipulation and mobilisation may or may not be effective for chronic neck pain.

In view of the research evidence not being specific to WAD and its inconclusive nature, questions were included in the Delphi process. Delphi findings indicate that, in the chronic stage, the following reduce pain:

- Manual mobilisation (*consensus* 78%)

- Combined manipulation and manual mobilisation (*consensus* 70%)

- Manipulation (*consensus* 59%).

Combined manipulation and manual mobilisation improves function (*consensus* 70%)

Manipulation and exercise is more effective than manipulation alone in:

- Improving function (*consensus* 89%)

- Reducing long term pain (*consensus* 85%)

- Patient satisfaction (*majority view* 74%).

Delphi findings were inconclusive on the relative benefits of the following in reducing pain:

- Manual mobilisation versus ice

- Manual mobilisation versus combined ice and TENS

- Manual mobilisation versus acupuncture

- Manual mobilisation versus a single manipulation.

Evidence Summary 34	Level
Manual therapy	
• Manual mobilisation may reduce pain (*consensus* 78%)	IV
• Combined manipulation and manual mobilisation may reduce pain (*majority view* 70%)	IV
• Manipulation may reduce pain (*majority view* 59%)	IV
• Combined manipulation and manual mobilisation may improve function (*majority view* 70%)	IV
• Manipulation and exercise may be more effective than manipulation alone in:	IV
improving function (*consensus* 89%)	IV
reducing long term pain (*consensus* 85%)	IV
patient satisfaction (*majority view* 74%)	IV

4.3.2 Exercise therapy

One RCT in people with chronic whiplash injuries by Fitz-Ritson[34] compared standard exercises (stretching, isometric, isokinetic) with 'phasic' exercises, consisting of rapid eye-hand-neck-arm movements. Both groups of people also received unspecified chiropractic treatment. The methodological quality of this study was poor (PEDro 3/10). It was not possible to tell if the randomisation process was concealed sufficiently as it was reported that people drew their group allocation from a box, without further details. Other serious flaws were that prognostic factors, such as age, gender, and the number of previous accidents in the two groups were not similar at the start of the study and outcome assessment was not blind to the treatment received. The percentage improvement in total average scores using the Neck Disability Index was 7.4% for the standard exercises and 48.3% for the 'phasic' exercise group after the eight weeks of treatment. These were both significantly different from baseline scores. This study did not directly compare the results from the two groups and did not describe the methods or results in detail.

A recent systematic review of exercise therapy in non-specific neck pain showed inconsistent evidence for the use of group exercise for chronic or frequent neck pain.[144] Evidence was found to support the use of proprioceptive exercises in reducing subjective pain and disability, although the evidence was conflicting for objective measures of function. There was also evidence to support the use of dynamic resisted strengthening exercises for the neck and shoulder. However, Delphi consensus was sought on these points because the evidence was not from a study involving people with WAD.

Another systematic review of rehabilitation interventions for neck pain[150] found two RCTs comparing group fitness classes versus unspecified control groups. No difference was found for either pain or sick leave at one or six months. An RCT with an active group receiving individual proprioceptive re-education showed that this relieved pain more than a waiting list control group.

Delphi findings contribute to the body of knowledge on the effects of exercise in the chronic stage as follows:

- Advice about coping strategies combined with exercise is more effective than exercise alone in returning to normal activity (*unanimity* 100%)

- Mobilising exercises are effective in reducing pain (*consensus* 96%)

- Exercises based on individual patient assessment are more effective than a generalised exercise programme in improving function (*consensus* 92%)

- Strengthening exercise is more effective than passive physiotherapy in improving function (*consensus* 76%)

- Proprioceptive exercise improves neck function (*majority view* 73%)

- Group exercise is effective in improving function (*majority view* 68%)

- Strengthening exercise is more effective than passive physiotherapy in reducing pain (*majority view* 62%)

- Extension retraction exercises are effective in improving neck function (*majority view* 58%)

- Standard exercise (stretching, isometric, isokinetic) is more effective than phasic exercise (rapid eye-hand-neck movements) in improving function (*majority view* 54%).

There is no Delphi evidence to suggest that strengthening exercises are more effective than either endurance training or body awareness training in reducing pain or in improving function.

Evidence Summary 35

Exercise therapy

	Level
• Advice about coping strategies combined with exercise is more effective than exercise alone in returning to normal activity (*unanimity* 100%)	IV
• Mobilising exercises are effective in reducing pain (*consensus* 96%)	IV
• Exercises based on individual patient assessment are more effective than a generalised exercise programme in improving function (*consensus* 92%)	IV
• Strengthening exercise is more effective than passive physiotherapy in improving function (*consensus* 76%)	IV
• Proprioceptive exercise improves neck function (*majority view* 73%)	IV
• Group exercise is effective in improving function (*majority view* 68%)	IV
• Strengthening exercise is more effective than passive physiotherapy in reducing pain (*majority view* 62%)	IV
• Extension retraction exercises are effective in improving neck function (*majority view* 58%)	IV
• Standard exercise (stretching, isometric, isokinetic) is more effective than phasic exercise (rapid eye-hand-neck movements) in improving function (*majority view* 54%)	IV

4.3.3 Physical agents (including electrotherapy)

No individual studies were found looking at the effects of physical agents in people with chronic whiplash injuries. A systematic review included an RCT that compared therapeutic ultrasound with placebo ultrasound but found no difference between them in relation to pain.[150] The same systematic review found no evidence relating to EMG biofeedback, massage, thermotherapy, electrical stimulation, or TENS in chronic neck pain.[150] Consensus evidence was not sought as this question arose after the Delphi questionnaire had been finalised and therefore was not included.

Evidence Summary 36

Physical agents

For non-specific neck pain:

	Level
• Therapeutic ultrasound is no more effective in reducing pain than placebo ultrasound.	Ia

4.3.4 Acupuncture

No studies were found that looked at the effectiveness of acupuncture for treating whiplash injuries alone. A systematic review by Smith et al.[153] investigating the effects of acupuncture on chronic neck and back pain included two RCTs of acupuncture for chronic neck pain, rated as low validity. One of these compared acupuncture with sham TENS and found no significant differences in pain at one week or 21-28 days after treatment. The other RCT compared traditional oriental meridian acupuncture with a delayed treatment control group and found a significant benefit for acupuncture (12/15 vs. 2/15 'improved'; relative benefit 6.0 (95%CI 1.6 to 22). Overall the review found no convincing evidence of pain relief by acupuncture for neck or back pain. Another systematic review[149] found two RCTs looking at people with mechanical neck pain: one acupuncture versus placebo and the other electro-acupuncture versus traction combined with short-wave diathermy. The trials did not support the use of acupuncture for mechanical neck pain..

A well-conducted RCT (Pedro 7/10) of people with chronic neck pain (due to fibromyalgia or whiplash) by Irnich et al (n=177) compared acupuncture with massage and with a control group that received sham laser acupuncture.[154] After one week, there was no significant difference between acupuncture and sham laser acupuncture, but motion related pain was significantly less in the acupuncture group than in the massage group. There were no statistically significant differences in pain related to motion and direction or health-related quality of life between the three treatments at three months.

Delphi findings were inconclusive in terms of whether acupuncture is more effective than either massage or sham acupuncture in reducing pain.

Evidence Summary 37   Level

Acupuncture

- Consensus neither supported nor refuted the use of acupuncture for people with chronic WAD.

For non-specific chronic neck pain:

- The effectiveness of acupuncture for chronic neck or back pain in reducing pain is inconclusive   Ia

- Acupuncture is as effective as massage and sham acupuncture for chronic neck and back pain   Ib

4.3.5 Multidisciplinary psychosocial rehabilitation

No reviews were found looking at the effectiveness of psychosocial interventions for chronic whiplash injuries and therefore evidence was sought from research on treatment for neck pain. A systematic review of multidisciplinary psychosocial rehabilitation in people with non-specific neck and/or shoulder pain[155] found two methodologically weak studies, only one of which was randomised. The non-randomised study showed no difference in effects of multidisciplinary active rehabilitation and traditional rehabilitation consisting of physiotherapy, rest and sick leave after 12 or 24 months of follow up. The RCT in the review found no differences in pain or functional status between a five-week in-patient multimodal cognitive behavioural therapy and a psychologist acting as a 'coach' to other health professionals, after the therapy ended or at six months.

A systematic overview of the evidence[14] found, in addition to the systematic review by Karjalainen,[155] two recent RCTs investigating the effectiveness of multimodal treatment of chronic non-specific neck pain. The overview found no consistent differences between multimodal cognitive behavioural therapy versus other treatments in level of pain or time taken off work. However in view of the absence of evidence from people with WAD this question was included in the Delphi questionnaire.

Delphi findings indicate that, in the chronic stage, multidisciplinary rehabilitation is more effective than traditional rehabilitation (physiotherapy, rest, sick leave) in improving function (*consensus* 78%).

Evidence Summary 38   Level

Multidisciplinary psychosocial rehabilitation

- Multidisciplinary rehabilitation is more effective than traditional rehabilitation (physiotherapy, rest, sick leave) in improving function (*consensus* 78%)   IV

For non-specific chronic neck pain:

- Intensive multidisciplinary programme with contact directly with a psychologist is no more effective than indirect psychological support from other trained health professionals for chronic neck pain.   Ib

Treatment recommendations for physiotherapy intervention for people with WAD in the chronic stage (i.e. more than 12 weeks after injury)

Grade

Manipulation and manual mobilisation

- The following should be considered for pain reduction: (ES 34)   C
  - Manual mobilisation
  - Manipulation
  - Combination of manipulation and manual mobilisation.

- Combination of manual mobilisation and manipulation should be considered to improve function.   C

Combining manipulation and exercise (ES 34)

- A combination of manipulation and exercise may be more effective than manipulation alone in: C
  - Reducing pain
  - Improving function
  - Increasing patient satisfaction

Exercise therapy (ES 35)

- Combined advice about coping strategies and exercise may be more effective than exercise alone in assisting people's return to normal activity.   C

- Mobilising exercises should be considered for the reduction of pain.   C

- Group exercise should be considered to improve function.   C

- Proprioceptive exercises should be considered to improve function.   C

- Strengthening exercises may be more effective than passive treatment in improving function and in reducing pain.   C

- Exercise based on individual assessment is likely to be more effective than general exercise in improving function.   C

- Standard exercise (stretching, isometric, isotonic) may be more effective than phasic exercise (rapid eye-hand-neck movements) in improving function.   C

- Extension retraction exercises could be considered to improve neck function.   C

Multidisciplinary psychosocial packages (ES 38)

- Multidisciplinary rehabilitation may be more effective than traditional rehabilitation (physiotherapy, rest, sick leave) in improving function.   C

Acupuncture (ES 37)

- There is no evidence to support or refute the use of acupuncture for people with WAD.

Physical agents (including electrotherapy) (ES 36)

- The use of the following cannot be supported or refuted:

  - Ultrasound
  - EMG biofeedback
  - Thermotherapy
  - Electrical stimulation
  - TENS
  - Massage

The GDG was keen to develop practical guidelines and to outline the kind of advice that is likely to be most useful to people with WAD. This information could not be drawn from the review carried out by the GDG, but a link is made to other work in the field. A recent systematic review of the literature has led to a framework for patient centred information and advice relating to WAD.[12] The emerging key messages from the review are:

- Serious physical injury is rare
- Reassurance about good prognosis is important
- Over medicalisation is detrimental
- Recovery is improved by early return to normal pre-accident activities, self-exercise and manual therapy
- Positive attitudes and beliefs are helpful in regaining activity levels
- Collars, rest and negative attitudes and beliefs delay recovery and contribute to chronicity.

These findings are published as *The Whiplash Book*.[78] This patient-focused booklet is recommended for use with for people with WAD, since it is based on consistent and reasonably robust evidence.

Evidence Summary 39	Level
Education and advice	
Summary statements about appropriate education and advice can be found in *The Whiplash Book*[78]	IV

Recommendations on education and advice that should be given to people with WAD (ES 39)	Grade
• Physical serious injury is rare	C
• Reassurance about good prognosis is important	C
• Over medicalisation is detrimental	C
• Recovery is improved by early return to normal pre-accident activities, self-exercise and manual therapy	C
• Positive attitudes and beliefs are helpful in regaining activity levels	C
• Collars, rest and negative attitudes and beliefs delay recovery and contribute to chronicity	C

Healthcare in the 21st century must be patient-centred. Physiotherapists need to be competent in communicating with patients and in understanding patients' needs and possess good education skills. An important aim of a physiotherapy intervention should be to enable patient empowerment and increase patient self-efficacy. These wider issues apply to the physiotherapy treatment of WAD.

4.5.1 Health care must be patient-centred

The NHS Plan clearly set out the need for more patient information, greater patient choice and a focus on patient-centred care.[156] This emphasis is also in evidence in the CSP's Standards of physiotherapy practice[123] and the Health Professions' Council Standards of Proficiency.[158]

Barr and Threlkeld see patients and clinicians as partners in the design of interventions which will achieve the best outcome for the particular person's lifestyle.[159] The models used in the establishment of a meaningful and effective partnership or therapeutic relationship have been described.[159, 160] The nature of the relationship between clinician and patient probably varies at different stages of treatment; sometimes the patient is more passive and at other times taking greater control. But the main aim of physiotherapy management is to encourage patients to take control of their own condition.

4.5.2 Communicating with patients and understanding their needs

Health Promotion experts have proposed a number of ways in which people can be helped to take more control of their health and grow in autonomy. Clinicians should understand patients' knowledge, beliefs, values and standards but also acknowledge that their own knowledge, values, beliefs and standards may differ significantly from the patients'.[161]

Trust and openness within the therapeutic relationship needs to be established from the start. It is important to ask patients what they are expecting from treatment because patients' expectations may differ from clinicians' expectations.[162] Patients should be given the opportunity to express their needs with regard to clinical management. Expressed needs are what patients say that they need. However patients may also have felt needs i.e. needs that they have identified themselves but that are limited by the patients' own knowledge of healthcare. Sometimes patients lack the motivation or assertiveness to express their felt needs and may need encouragement from clinicians. Evidence is growing that patients who are well informed about their treatment and the reasons for it, and who are involved in decisions, have better outcomes than those who do not share in the decision making process.[163] At the same time therapists may not be taking full advantage of patients' potential for participating in their own care, e.g. in goal setting.[164]

Good communication leads to patient empowerment, enhanced quality of care, improved satisfaction and better health outcomes. Professional practice should be modified in response to people's needs.[165] Communication is enhanced if the clinician speaks slowly and deliberately, keeps questions short and asks one question at a time. Good listening skills are essential[166] and clinicians need good interpersonal skills to pick up nuances from unspoken words or gestures.

4.5.3 Clinicians should possess good education skills

Clinicians' educational skills are vital to the therapist-patient partnership and in helping people to empower themselves and develop self-efficacy. Physiotherapists treating people with WAD are generally dealing with adult learners thus the principles described in Knowles' *Theory of Adult Learning*[167] will apply. Adults see themselves as self directed and responsible individuals in terms of learning. They possess a wealth of experience which is a resource for their learning. Adult learners are motivated to learn when they perceive the learning activity is directly related to their own personal circumstances and needs. They tend to focus on problem solving rather than abstract content or theory.[167] Many factors affect learning[168] but one of the strongest factors is learning styles which are related to personality.[169] It is important for clinicians to reflect on their own preferred learning style before engaging with patient education. This will make them sensitive to the fact that patients will have varied learning styles. Ewles and Simnett[161] have identified a number of principles for patient education:

1. Say important things first, people will remember best what was said first

2. Stress and repeat key points, emphasise the important points, repetition helps

3. Give specific precise advice related to people's own physical and social circumstances

4. Structure information, give people headings and deliver material under these headings

5. Avoid jargon, long words and long sentences

6. Use visual aid wherever possible e.g. leaflets, handouts, models, videos and written instructions

7. Avoid saying too much, only two or three key points will be remembered from each session

8. Ensure your advice is relevant and realistic with the person's lifestyle by discussing their needs with them

9. Ask for feedback from patients to assess their understanding either formally or informally; choose an assessment appropriate to patients' own learning style.

When teaching practical skills three stages have been recommended: a demonstration by the clinician, a rehearsal by the patient observed by the clinician, and practice by the patient alone but observed on a regular basis by the clinician.[161] Moore et al give further details on facilitating learning.[168]

4.5.4   Patient empowerment and self-efficacy

Empowerment has been defined as the process of enabling or imparting power transfer from one individual to another.[170] Empowerment should be seen as the result of an established therapeutic relationship, in other words it is a helping process which enables individuals to change a situation giving them the skill and resources and opportunities to do so. It embodies partnership; it aims to develop a positive belief in self and the future and encompasses mutual decision-making. It also gives individuals i.e. patients the freedom to make choices and accept responsibility for those choices and it recognises that power originates from self-esteem.

A further concept gaining popularity in healthcare systems across the world is self-efficacy. Self-efficacy enables a bridge to be built between the person (the patient) and their own social world, this implies that the individual must make changes to their behaviour in order to maintain or improve their health or disability status.[171] Self-efficacy generally relates to an individual's confidence in their ability to make a specific change in their behaviour which can be very relevant in terms of people with chronic pain.[172] Self help groups and peer support can be highly instrumental in improving and increasing self-efficacy and have been used extensively in the management of rheumatoid arthritis in the USA and South Africa and the concept is spreading rapidly into other countries.

Summary of the recommendations

Using these recommendations

These recommendations indicate best physiotherapy practice for adults who have experienced whiplash injuries. However, treatment cannot be prescriptive and should always follow individual assessment. **A** grade recommendations are based on findings of controlled trial(s), **B** grade recommendations on other well conducted studies, **C** grade recommendations on expert opinion and good practice points on the expertise of the Guidelines Development Group (GDG) (see section 2.7 and Appendix A)

Mechanism of injury (ES 1)

Physiotherapists should be aware of theories that are developing to explain the mechanism of whiplash injury in order that they can relate the site of injury to the person's symptoms and plan their physiotherapy management   **B**

Classification (ES 2)

The Quebec Task Force classification should be used by physiotherapists for WAD with grade II subdivided into IIa and IIb, in order to assist with diagnosis and prognosis.   **Good practice point**

Recovery (ES 3)

Physiotherapists should advise people with WAD that they are very likely to recover.   **C**

Risk factors that may influence prognosis

Information should be sought in order that risk factors can be identified at the assessment stage as they can adversely affect prognosis.

At the time of injury, the following factors indicate that a poor prognosis is likely (ES 4)

- Relatively low weight of person's vehicle compared with other vehicle involved   **B**
- Poor headrest position (i.e. not level with the top of the head, not close to the back of the head)   **C**
- Rear end collisions where the person is looking to one side.   **C**

The following pre-existing factors indicate a poorer prognosis is likely (ES 5)

- Pre-trauma neck ache   **B**
- Pre-existing degenerative changes   **C**
- Low level of job satisfaction   **C**
- Pre-trauma headaches   **C**

The following post-injury factors indicate that a poorer prognosis is likely (ES 6)

- High initial pain intensity   **B**
- Headache for more than six months following injury   **C**
- Neurological signs present after injury   **C**

Barriers to recovery

Psychosocial barriers to recovery (ES 7)

- Compensation issues may not be a barrier to recovery from WAD   **B**

- Physiotherapists should be aware of the wide range of psychosocial barriers to recovery:　　　　　　　C
  · high fear of pain and movement
  · low self-efficacy
  · severe anxiety
  · severe depression
  · low pain locus of control
  · high use of passive coping strategies
  · chronic widespread pain
  · high tendency to catastrophise
  · problems in relationships with others
  · a series of previously failed treatments
  · non-compliance with treatment and advice
  · unrealistic expectations of treatment
  · inability to work because of the pain
  · negative expectations of treatment
  · poor understanding of the healing mechanism
  · failure of the physiotherapist to meet an individual person's needs
  · poor clinical reasoning by the physiotherapist

- Physiotherapists should assess for psychosocial barriers at all stages after injury　　　　C

- Ongoing moderate to severe symptoms six months after injury are likely to be associated with post traumatic stress syndrome　　　　C

Occupational barriers to recovery (ES 8)

Physiotherapists should be aware that perception of work and job context and working conditions may be barriers to recovery　　　　C

Range of possible symptoms encountered with WAD (ES 9 and section 3.5)

Physiotherapists should be aware that the symptoms of WAD can include: neck pain, headache, shoulder and arm pain, generalised hypersensitivity, paraesthesia and muscle weakness, temporomandibular joint pain and dysfunction, visual disturbance, impairment of the proprioceptive control of head and neck position and impaired cognitive function　　　　B

Physiotherapy assessment and examination of people with WAD

Valid consent (ES 10)

Valid consent should be sought and recorded in line with national standards and guidance, and local organisational policy　　　　C

Access to physiotherapy service (ES 11, 12)

Physiotherapists should prioritise entry into the physiotherapy service by:

- Screening individual people　　　　C

- Providing a physiotherapy service in the accident and emergency department **C**

- Assessing individual people by telephone　　　　C

Physiotherapists should prioritise people who:

- Find their activities of daily living disrupted as a result of WAD　　　　C

- Are unable to work as a result of WAD　　　　C

- Have a more recent injury　　　　C

Subjective assessment (ES 13)

A thorough subjective assessment is essential to help plan subsequent examination and treatment.　　　　**Good practice point**

Serious pathology (red flags) (ES 14)

- People with WAD must be screened for red flags.   **Good practice point**

- People with bilateral paraesthesia, gait disturbance, spastic paresis, positive Lhermittes sign, hyper reflexia, nerve root signs at more than two adjacent levels, progressively worsening neurological signs, symptoms of upper cervical instability, non-mechanical pain which is unremitting and severe must be referred immediately to the nearest accident and emergency department.   **Good practice point**

- People with positive stress tests of the cranio-vertebral joints, vertebral column malignancy or infection, a past history of cancer, rheumatoid arthritis, long-term steroid use, osteoporosis, systemically unwell generally, structural deformity, other conditions and syndromes associated with instability or hypermobility should be treated with caution.   **Good practice point**

The physical examination (ES 15)

- Joint instability testing should only be conducted by a specially trained physiotherapist   **Good practice point**

- Cervical manipulation and pre-manipulative testing techniques should be avoided for people with WAD   **Good practice point**

- Physiotherapists need to know when special tests and investigations are indicated and how to carry out the tests or refer people appropriately   **Good practice point**

- **People with WAD presenting with signs and symptoms of instability must immediately be referred for further investigation**   **Good practice point**

- Inexperienced physiotherapists must know when to ask advice from senior staff   **Good practice point**

Defining the aims of physiotherapy treatment (ES 16)

Although treatment is tailored to individual needs general aims of physiotherapy treatment should be to:

- Improve function   **C**
- Facilitate empowerment of the person with WAD   **C**
- Return the person to normal activity/work   **C**
- Relieve symptoms   **C**

Advising on pain relief (ES 17)

- Physiotherapists should refer to local guidelines for prescription of analgesia   **Good practice point**

- Where guidelines do not exist physiotherapists and people with WAD should seek appropriate medical advice   **Good practice point**

Treatment recommendations for physiotherapy intervention for WAD in the acute stage (zero to two weeks after injury)

Grade

Soft collars

- The use of soft collars is not recommended (ES 18) C

Manual mobilisation

- Manual mobilisation should be considered for the reduction of neck pain in the initial stages (ES 21) B
- Manual mobilisation should be considered to increase neck range of movement (ES 21) C
- Manual mobilisation should be considered to improve function (ES 21) C
- Soft tissue techniques should be considered for the reduction of pain (ES 19) C

Exercise therapy

- Active exercise should be used to reduce pain (ES 19 and 22) A
- Active exercise for pain reduction should be started within 4 days of injury (ES 22) A
- An active exercise programme devised for each individual following assessment should be considered for the reduction of pain (ES 19) C

Education and advice

- Education on self-management should be provided, to reduce patients' symptoms (ES 24) A
- Returning to normal activities as soon as possible should be encouraged (ES 20) A
- Providing education about the origin of the pain should be considered for reducing pain (ES 19) C
- Providing advice about coping strategies may be helpful for the reduction of pain (ES 19) C
- Relaxation should be considered for reducing pain (ES 19) C

Physical agents (including electrotherapy)

- The use of TENS should be considered for reducing pain (ES 19) C
- The following are unlikely to be effective in reducing pain: (ES 19) C
  · Traction
  · Infrared light
  · Interferential therapy
  · Ultrasound treatment
  · Laser treatment
- There is insufficient evidence to support or refute the use of the following (ES 19)
  · Massage C
  · Acupuncture C
  · PEMT **Good practice point**

Treatment recommendations for physiotherapy intervention for WAD in the sub acute stage (i.e. more than 2 weeks and up to 12 weeks after injury)

Grade

Manipulation and manual mobilisation

- Combined manipulation and manual mobilisation should be considered for reducing pain (ES 26)

C

- Combined manipulation and manual mobilisation should be considered for improving function (ES 26)

C

- The risk of serious adverse events from cervical manipulation may be increased after whiplash injury (ES 27)

Good practice point

Exercise therapy

- There is unlikely to be any benefit in including kinaesthetic exercise in a programme of functional improvement exercise (ES 28)

B

- Muscle retraining including deep neck flexor activity may be effective in improving function (ES 33)

C

Multimodal packages

- A multimodal programme (including postural training, manual techniques and psychological support) should be used to reduce pain and speed return to work (ES 29)

A

Acupuncture

- The use of acupuncture cannot be supported or refuted (ES 30)

C

Education and advice (ES 31)

- Education should be considered for the improvement of neck function (ES 31)

C

- Advice about coping strategies should be considered, to enable people to return to normal activities (ES 31)

C

Physical agents (including electrotherapy)

The following treatments could be considered for the reduction of pain: (ES 33)

C

- TENS
- Massage
- Soft tissue techniques

The following treatments are unlikely to reduce neck pain:

C

- Traction (ES 32)
- Infrared light (ES 33)
- Interferential therapy (ES 33)
- Laser treatment (ES 33)
- Ultrasound (ES 33)

Treatment recommendations for physiotherapy intervention for people   Grade
with WAD in the chronic stage (i.e. more than 12 weeks after injury)

Manipulation and manual mobilisation

- The following should be considered for pain reduction: (ES 34)   C
  · Manual mobilisation
  · Manipulation
  · Combination of manipulation and manual mobilisation.

- Combination of manual mobilisation and manipulation should be considered
  to improve function.   C

Combining manipulation and exercise (ES 34)

- A combination of manipulation and exercise may be more effective than manipulation alone in: C
  · Reducing pain
  · Improving funciton
  · Increasing patient satisfaction

Exercise therapy (ES 35)

- Combined advice about coping strategies and exercise may be more effective than exercise
  alone in assisting people's return to normal activity   C

- Mobilising exercises should be considered for the reduction of pain   C

- Group exercise should be considered to improve function   C

- Proprioceptive exercises should be considered to improve function   C

- Strengthening exercises may be more effective than passive treatment in improving function
  and in reducing pain   C

- Exercise based on individual assessment is likely to be better than general exercise in
  improving function   C

- Standard exercise (stretching, isometric, isotonic) may be more effective than phasic
  exercise (rapid eye-hand-neck movements) in improving function   C

- Extension retraction exercises could be considered to improve neck function   C

Multidisciplinary psychosocial packages (ES 38)

- Multidisciplinary rehabilitation may be more effective than traditional rehabilitation
  (physiotherapy, rest, sick leave) in improving function   C

Acupuncture (ES 37)

- There is no evidence to support or refute the use of acupuncture for people with WAD.

Physical agents (including electrotherapy) (ES 36)

- The use of the following cannot be supported or refuted:
  · Ultrasound
  · EMG biofeedback
  · Thermotherapy
  · Electrical stimulation
  · TENS
  · Massage

Recommendations on education and advice that should be given to people with WAD (ES 39)	Grade
• Physical serious injury is rare	C
• Reassurance about good prognosis is important	C
• Over medicalisation is detrimental	C
• Recovery is improved by early return to normal pre-accident activities, self-exercise and manual therapy	C
• Positive attitudes and beliefs are helpful in regaining activity levels	C
• Collars, rest and negative attitudes and beliefs delay recovery and contribute to chronicity	C

Research recommendations

Questions for future research

The gaps in the available research evidence that have been identified in the development of these guidelines provide a useful basis for considering appropriate research questions, for which funding can be sought. As there is little definitive evidence for physiotherapy for people with WAD there is a wide range of research recommendations.

6.1 Physiotherapy treatment modalities for people with WAD

- Do soft collars relieve pain compared with advice from a physiotherapist?
- Does manual mobilisation relieve pain compared with advice from a physiotherapist?
- Does manipulation relieve pain compared with advice from a physiotherpist?
- What is the cost-effectiveness of soft collars or manual mobilisation or manipulation, compared with advice from a physiotherapist?
- Does a cognitive behavioural intervention speed return to normal activity compared with advice from a physiotherapist?

Similar questions might be asked of other physiotherapy interventions eg TENS, massage, soft tissue techniques.

6.2 Service development, prioritising treatment and the natural history of WAD

- What is the optimal treatment period for people with WAD?
- Do between four and six visits to a physiotherapist speed return to normal function compared with one session of advice from a physiotherapist?
- What is normal versus delayed recovery time for people with WAD?
- What factors can be used to predict outcome?
- Which biopsychosocial factors are predictive of a successful treatment outcome?
- Does early physiotherapy intervention in the accident and emergency department speed return to normal activity compared with later treatment in the physiotherapy department?
- At which stage of WAD is physiotherapy most effective i.e. acute, subacute or chronic?

6.3 Education and advice for people with WAD

For people with WAD:

- Which exercises should be recommended for WAD?
- Does an individualised exercise programme speed return to normal activity compared with generalised group exercise?
- At what stages and at what frequency is exercise most useful?
- Does an exercise programme given in the first three days since injury speed return to normal activity compared with an exercise programme given two weeks or more after injury?
- What advice should be given to people with WAD?

- Does implementation of these guidelines in a physiotherapy department speed patients' return to normal activity, compared with before the guidelines' implementation?

Outcome measures relevant to the treatment of people with WAD

Physiotherapists need to know whether treatment has made a difference to people with WAD. This will help in understanding the nature of WAD and assist in decision making. CSP core standard six [123] indicates that a published, standardised, valid, reliable and responsive outcome measure should be used to evaluate the change in people's health status after physiotherapy intervention. There are several measures that clinicians might consider to evaluate treatment outcome for people with WAD [173] but evidence suggests that physiotherapists may have difficulty finding and choosing outcome measures. [174]

This section identifies a number of measures that might be of use to clinicians. There are many factors to take into account e.g. the nature of the service, the outcome measures already used and the aims of the intervention. The measures suggested here are not recommendations. Each measure should be appraised for validity, reliability and practicality in a particular setting. A range of tools is suggested but it is for practitioners to decide on the aspects of outcome that should be measured.

7.1 Pain

The Visual Analogue Scale (VAS)

The VAS measures intensity of pain and is not disease specific. [175] The patient is asked to indicate where, on a 100mm straight line, best describes their pain, with one end representing 'no pain' and the other end the 'worst pain possible'. Reliability and validity is established. It usually takes about a minute to complete and is extremely straightforward. Permission to print this scale is unnecessary as it is in the public domain. It is available from: http://www.britishpainsociety.org/pain_scales.html

7.2 Function

The Neck Disability Index

The Neck Disability Index measures function and is derived from the Oswestry Low Back Pain Index. It includes questions about pain, headaches, ability to concentrate, sleep patterns, lifting abilities, work, car driving, hobbies or sport or recreation, activities of daily living and reading. [176] It takes a few minutes to complete and has demonstrated clinical validity [177,178] in addition to reliability, sensitivity to severity of condition and changes after intervention. [177-179] It is recommended that users contact the authors to ensure that they are using the most recent version.

7.3 Return to usual activities

The Physiotherapy Specific Function Scale

This tool measures return to usual activities. [180] It is recommended that users contact the authors to ensure that they are using the most recent version.

The Measure Yourself Medical Outcome Profile (MYMOP)

The MYMOP was devised to measure patient generated outcomes in primary care and has been demonstrated to be valid and more sensitive to change than the SF-36 health survey.[181] It is not disease specific and is a practical tool for use in clinical practice. It has four items; the first two relate to two symptoms that are particularly problematic, the third to a functional activity and the fourth to general feeling of wellbeing. It is scored on a seven point Likert scale; the MYMOP profile score is the mean difference in the four items. The measure is in the public domain and so it is unnecessary to gain permission to use it. Full details can be found from: http://www.hsrc.ac.uk/mymop
(Accessed 9th June 2005)

The Tampa Scale for Kineisiophobia (TSK)

The TSK is a 17-item questionnaire that measures people's fear of movement/(re)injury.[182] People rate each of the questions on a four-point Likert scale with scoring alternatives ranging from 'strongly disagree' to 'strongly agree'. The scores on items four, eight, 12, and 16 are reversed. Total scores range from 17 to 68, with higher scores being indicative of a higher fear of movement/re) injury. The Dutch version of the TSK has good reliability and validity.[183,184] Recent findings have also shown that the English version of the TSK possesses good reliability and validity.[185, 186]

The Short Form 36 Health Survey Questionnaire (SF-36)

This is well established as a valid and reliable general measure of health status. It gives an indication of quality of life and covers functional status, wellbeing, overall evaluation of health and change in health. Users may consider whether the shorter versions i.e. the SF-12 or the SF-8 may be more appropriate for their purposes. Permission to use this tool in clinical practice needs to be gained from the web site where an online licence application form can be completed: http://www.sf-36.com
(Accessed 9th June 2005)

Patient satisfaction can be evaluated using the Patient Feedback Questionnaire, part of the clinical audit tools to support implementation of the CSPs Standards of Physiotherapy Practice. The clinical audit tool [187] has been developed to assist physiotherapists in providing the best possible service. Patients are asked a series of questions including how long they waited for an appointment, how much input they had in deciding their treatment plan, how sensitive physiotherapists were to their fears and anxieties, and how they felt about their discharge. Most questions involve ticking a box but people are invited to comment on some issues. The tool can be downloaded free of charge from:
http://www.csp.org.uk/effectivepractice/standards/publications.cfm?id=210 (Accessed 9th June 2005)

Anxiety and depression

The Hospital Anxiety and Depression Scale (HADS)

The HADS[188] is a 14-item scale that assesses anxiety (seven items) and depression (seven items). The scale does not assess severe psychopathology and might, therefore, be more acceptable to people with chronic pain.[189] The HADS is also thought to be more sensitive to mild forms of psychiatric disorders, thus avoiding the 'floor effect', where respondents cluster around the lowest possible score and change is harder to detect, and which is frequently observed when psychiatric questionnaires are used for people with chronic pain.[189] All items are scored on a four-point scale from zero to three. Both the anxiety and depression subscales have established validity and reliability.[190–192] There is no single, generally accepted cut-off score for the HADS. In the original study two cut-off scores for both subscales: 7/8 for possible and 10/11 for probable anxiety or depression (with ranges of 0–21 for each subscale) were recommended.[188] The scale can be ordered from:
http://www.nfer-nelson.co.uk/catalogue/catalogue_detail.asp?catid=98&id=1125
(Accessed 9th June 2005)

Self-efficacy

The Chronic Pain Self-efficacy Scale (CPSS)

The CPSS[193] is a 22-item measure containing three subscales, which assess a person's (a) self-efficacy for pain management (five-items), (b) self-efficacy for physical function (nine-items), and (c) self-efficacy for coping with symptoms (eight-items). The measure possesses good reliability and validity.[193] The scale appears as an Appendix to the cited paper and thus it is freely available.

Delphi findings and GDG advice

Delphi findings indicate that the following are likely to be useful outcome measures:

- **For pain:** The visual analogue scale (*consensus* 93%)

- **For function:** The neck disability index (*consensus* 78%)

- **For quality of life:** The SF-36 (*majority view* 58%)

- **For anxiety and depression:** The hospital anxiety and depression scale (*majority view* 54%)

The GDG felt that many clinicians needed greater awareness of the range of outcome measures available. For these reasons the GDG advise that any of the outcome measures in section 7could be considered for people with WAD.

The GDG, using informal consensus methods, suggest that the following tools may be useful in measuring outcome of WAD:

- **For return to usual activities:** The physiotherapy specific functional scale

- **For a patient centred measure:** Measure yourself medical outcome profile (MYMOP)

- **For fear of movement:** The Tampa scale of kinesiophobia (TSK)

- **For patient satisfaction:** The CSP's clinical audit tool, The patient feedback questionnaire

- **For self-efficacy:** The chronic pain self-efficacy scale (CPSS)

Legal issues

Patients requiring legal advice may obtain details of qualified solicitors who deal with personal injury cases from the Law Society tel. 0207 242 1222 web site www.lawsociety.org.uk (Accessed 9th June 2005) or www.solicitors-online.com (Accessed 9th June 2005).

Physiotherapists may be required to produce records or prepare a report for legal purposes in connection with people's WAD injuries. They should follow their organisational policy and procedures and also contact the CSP for advice. The information paper Reports for Legal Purposes (PA1) can be downloaded from www.csp.org.uk/libraryandinformation/publications/view.cfm?id=153 (Accessed 9th June 2005).[194] Some key points are outlined below.

- The solicitor should confirm the request in writing and state that a fee will be payable

- The patient's written consent to the release of information contained in the notes should accompany the request

- Physiotherapists should ensure that local organisational protocols are followed

- Junior physiotherapists should seek assistance from their clinical supervisors

- Physiotherapy reports should contain information under the following headings:
  · history
  · examination and treatment
  · future care and prognosis
  · conclusion

- Physiotherapists must separate information in the report into three categories: information that is reported to them by people with WAD, observable facts and professional opinions

- Inexperienced physiotherapists should seek advice where necessary.

9

Implementation

Implementation is defined as the systematic introduction of an innovation, a plan or a change of proven value.[195] Research findings will only influence clinical practice if that knowledge is translated into action.[196] Policy-makers, managers, professional body representatives, educators and managers can all promote the use of guidelines but in practice it is clinicians and their patients who implement recommendations. Developing and publishing good quality guidelines is not a guarantee for improved clinical practice.[197] Clinicians may find the use of guidelines inconvenient, time consuming and in conflict with their own clinical experience. In addition, national and local guidelines may be inconsistent and this can lead to confusion and frustration.[198] These guidelines for the treatment of WAD are therefore likely to present challenges to clinical physiotherapists seeking to implement them.

Over the past decade, there has been an increase in the understanding of the many factors (social, behavioural and organisational) which act as barriers to change. Some factors influence the behaviour of health care professionals e.g. the organisation, the system, peer groups, senior colleagues, and individual preference and opinion. All of these factors mean that implementation of guideline recommendations is a complex issue. Implementation strategies are necessary to ensure that guidelines enhance knowledge, and change values, beliefs, attitudes and clinicians' perceptions.[199] Currently there is little evidence to direct us to the most appropriate dissemination and implementation strategy for clinical guidelines. However, appraisal of the common barriers and facilitators to change are useful starting points.

9.2 Potential barriers and facilitators

A guidelines implementation strategy should seek to address known key barriers, maximise identified facilitators, be adequately planned and well monitored. Many important barriers have been identified.[196] Factors which in some circumstances may be perceived as barriers to change can sometimes act as levers for change e.g. patients' expectations and opinion leaders' views.[196] The following provides a brief summary of some key barriers and facilitators and how they can be applied to theseguidelines.

9.2.1 Knowledge barriers

Knowledge of the existence of guidelines and thus the recommendations made may be limited.[200] In a recent survey, physiotherapists who were questioned about methods of dissemination, suggested that the CSP should raise awareness of important publications.[201]

The CSP promotes an awareness of the availability of the guidelines to all members through, for example:

- Articles in 'Frontline' and other relevant publications
- Promoting the guidelines at CSP congresses
- Liasing with relevant clinical interest groups
- Liasing with universities to influence undergraduate and postgraduate students.

9.2.2 Organisational barriers (including time)

Time limitations and difficulties in communication and collaboration with other healthcare practitioners have been identified as barriers to the use of guidelines within physiotherapy.[195,200] Clinicians need time to appraise guidelines, to discuss the recommendations and consider the implications of implementation. Practice setting may be important e.g. physiotherapists working in isolation in community clinics or private practice may experience inadequate peer support and access to information.[201] There are important differences in the needs and perspectives of clinicians and their managers in applying guidelines.[201] Locally, it will be important that managers and clinicians support activities such as those set out below, to facilitate implementation:

- Discussion groups to break down barriers across different practice settings (including private practice)[200]

- Identification and recognition of the perspectives of both clinicians and managers

- Educational support and outreach with protected time for these activities.[200]

9.2.3 Cost and access

Although physiotherapists may be aware of the existence of guidelines, studies have shown they have difficulty in obtaining copies, or they may be frustrated by sharing one copy amongst many colleagues.[201] The cost of guidelines can also contribute to difficulties with access.

The CSP currently makes available:

- Free summaries of guidelines which are widely disseminated

- Access to the full guidelines on the CSP web-site with free downloadable copies.

To overcome cost and access barriers the CSP is also considering:

- Producing the full guidelines on CD-ROM.

9.2.4 Practitioner factors

These include the beliefs and attitudes of clinicians, the skills of individual clinicians, the influence of opinion leaders and the local experience of adapting practice to national guidelines. Some clinicians will hold beliefs that differ to the guidelines recommendations and/or may adhere to traditional or alternative practices. The implementation strategy will need to address these issues. A frequently reported barrier to the implementation of guidelines relates to a lack of knowledge or skills in the target group of clinicians.[195,200]

These barriers may be addressed by:

- Continuing professional development and education

- Making a strong link between other initiatives within the profession, for example evidence-based practice and to other national guidelines.

Guidelines recommendations can identify areas where individual clinicians need additional education and training. A qualitative study identified several physiotherapists who felt that they had insufficient knowledge and skill in using cognitive-behavioural principles or manipulation in managing people with back pain.[200] In addition, physiotherapists have reported a lack of knowledge in applying behavioural principles to exercise therapy.[195]

9.2.5 Patient expectations

It is becoming increasingly clear that patients' beliefs and expectations of treatment influence treatment outcome.[202, 203] Patients' expectations may act as a barrier to guidelines implementation as many patients may have preferences for interventions now considered outdated or ineffective. This highlights the importance of dealing with patient expectations as part of the decision-making process when using clinical guidelines in practice. Implementation for these guidelines may need to include education and role-play on incorporating patients' preferences and expectations into decision-making.

9.3 Interpreting the implications of guidelines recommendations

Guidelines recommendations are based on consensus in addition to scientific evidence.[204] Therefore recommendations are influenced by both the research evidence surrounding the efficacy of different interventions and also by the views and opinions of the GDG membership.[204] When translating evidence into clinically relevant recommendations, many factors play a role and these factors can vary locally and nationally (Table 9.1). It is likely that nationally developed guidelines will undergo a level of local adaptation before they are implemented.

9.4 The challenge of implementing guidelines

Research is needed to:

- Study the effectiveness of guidelines implementation strategies
- Demonstrate that implementing recommendations improves patient outcomes.

Studies in this area have been conducted by other professional groups [205, 206] and it is beginning to be addressed by physiotherapists in the UK.[207]

Systematic reviews show that information transfer is essential to the process of implementation; practitioners need to know about the guidelines. However passive methods of disseminating and implementing guidelines e.g. publication in professional journals or mailing targeted healthcare professionals, rarely changes professional behaviour.[208–210] Rather, multiple interventions are more likely to change practice[210] and these are summarised below (Table 9.1).

| Table 9.1 | Summary of the effectiveness of interventions to promote implementation |

Level of effectiveness	Strategy
Consistently effective	Educational outreach visits
	Reminders (computerised or manual)
	Multifaceted interventions (combining two or more of the following: audit and feedback, reminders, local consensus process and marketing)
	Interactive educational meetings (participation of clinicians in workshops that include discussions or practice)
Mixed effects	Audit and feedback (any summary of clinical performance)
	Local opinion leaders (use of 'expert' clinicians nominated by their colleagues as educationally influential)
	Local consensus process (inclusion of participating providers in discussion to ensure agreed approach to management of the clinical problem)
	Patient-mediated interventions (any intervention aimed at changing the performance of clinicians where specific information was sought from or given to patients)
Little or no effect	Educational materials (distribution of published or printed recommendations for clinical care, including clinical practice guidelines, audio-visual materials and electronic publications)
	Didactic educational meetings (lectures)

Adapted from Bero et al[209] in Haines and Donald[196]

Active strategies for implementing and assessing the effectiveness of new guidelines are essential. Suggested strategies include the use of reminders of guidelines' availability and locally held interactive educational meetings about the guidelines' content.[209] Improved adherence to guidelines for back pain management by physiotherapists (n=113) was demonstrated when an active implementation strategy was used.[195] Physiotherapists' knowledge of guideline recommendations has been improved by education, discussion, role-playing, feedback and reminders.[211, 212]

9.5 Methods of dissemination and implementation of these guidelines

Various methods will be used to disseminate the WAD guidelines. These will include:

- Articles to promote the guidelines in 'Frontline'
- Press releases to relevant professional bodies and other organisations
- The guidelines will be available to download from the CSP web site
- Printed copies will be available for purchase through the CSP
- Promoting the guidelines at the CSP Congress.

9.6 Implementation/audit pack

An audit/implementation pack will be developed by the CSP to support implementation of these guidelines.

10

Using the guidelines in clinical practice

This section considers the theory of reflective practice and applies this theory to the WAD guidelines. The accompanying 'reflective practice record sheet' (Appendix J) may be used by physiotherapy practitioners as part of their continuing professional development. The intention is to suggest a starting point for applying the guidelines to clinical practice.

10.1 Why reflect?

As practitioners we make decisions on the basis of:

- Formal information gained by asking questions, focusing on observable features and balancing probabilities amidst a degree of uncertainty, for example information from high quality clinical research and from patients

- Less formal information, drawn from our personal assumptions and intuition about the nuances of situations.

When trying to describe or justify our clinical decisions, or explain our development needs, it can be difficult to distinguish between intuitive thoughts and conscious pattern recognition, based on previously encountered similar situations.

Reflecting on our practice alone and with our colleagues can help us to

- Think about our **formal decision-making**; what we do well as practitioners and what areas need improvement

- Assess our level of self-awareness, examine the assumptions that underlie our thoughts and understand the contribution they make to our decisions – **intuitive decision-making**

- Confirm our own values and confront ethical dilemmas in our practice so we become empowered to take action – **ethical decision-making**.

These areas and their overlap are illustrated in figure 10.1.

| Figure 10.1 | Overlap between reflective activities |

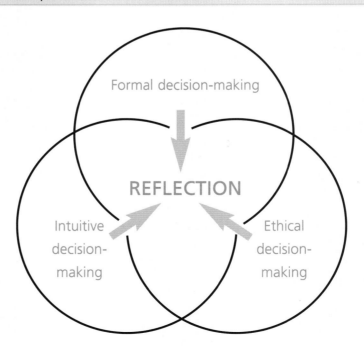

Finding a focus for reflection on practice can be difficult. Section 4 of the WAD guidelines provides a useful framework by:

1. Raising key questions about WAD-related practice

2. Identifying two key areas for consideration in relation to each question:

    *   what is the **evidence** and where do gaps in the evidence exist?

    *   what **recommendations** will help ensure best practice in the current state of knowledge about WAD?

    But it is also useful to add a third key area for consideration when reflecting:

    *   What is the **clinical relevance** across a broad range of factors – assessment, intervention, psychosocial factors, medico legal issues?

Figure 10.2 illustrates how this framework links to the reflective process described above.

Figure 10.2   Linking reflection to the WAD guideline

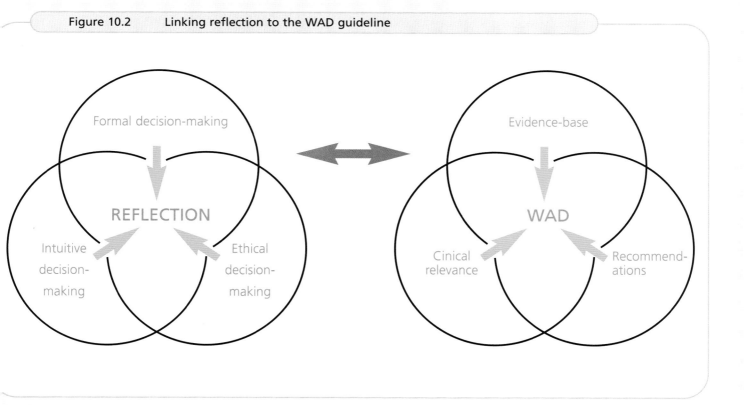

A **reflective practice record sheet** to help summarise your reflective practice in relation to WAD is included with these guidelines, in Appendix J.

1. The record sheet starts with a description of a whiplash related **practice-based event**. This might have occurred, for example, during an assessment or intervention, a psychosocial interaction or an administrative process. It might have involved any or all of the three types of decision making described on the left of figure 11.2.

2. Think generally about how you responded. Describe your objective thoughts and actions as well as your subjective feelings.

3. Try to explain why you responded as you did.

4. Next, set this experience in the WAD framework by considering what clinical question/s it might be linked to, for example 'what are the symptoms of WAD?' or 'what is the prognosis and natural history of WAD?' (see the clinical questions, section 2.2 and sections 3.6 and 3.7)

Go on to consider what issues your experience seems to raise in relation to the three key elements above.

5. **Evidence-base:** did your experience confirm existing evidence or demonstrate a gap? Have you any thoughts about how such a gap could be addressed in the context of your own or others' practice?

6. **Clinical relevance:** how did your experience demonstrate the clinical relevance of the identified question/s? Perhaps it called their relevance into question?

7. **Recommendations:** to what extent did your response conform to expected good practice as defined in the WAD guidelines? Does it suggest any additions or amendments to the recommendations?

Now examine what the event has revealed about your own personal development in terms of:

8. **Formal decision-making:** is there a development need? What are your strengths?

9. **Intuitive decision-making:** how well were you able to articulate your intuitive thoughts? Has the event revealed anything about your assumptions and level of self-awareness?

10. **Ethical decision-making:** did you feel any conflict of values? How well did you deal with it?

11. Finally, ask yourself, is this a recurring scenario? In other words, have you completed several reflective practice record sheets that describe similar events and issues? Have others recounted similar experiences when you have shared your reflections with your colleagues? If so, are there any **policy implications** that ought to be discussed and disseminated to a wider audience across the department or trust?

Links with other guidelines

11.1 Guidelines for the use of radiological investigations

The Royal College of Radiologists has published guidelines for making he best use of a department of clinical radiology.[135] Extracts from this document, relating to diagnostic imaging of the cervical spine, can be found in Appendix H.

11.2 Other guidelines about WAD

- Guidelines for the management of whiplash-associated disorders (2001) Motor Accidents Authority, Sydney, NSW.[213]

- Physiotherapy in common neck pain and whiplash (2003) Agencie Nationale d'Acreditation et d'Evaluation en Sante. (Translation from French). [214]

- Clinical practice guidelines for physical therapy in patients with whiplash-associated disorders on Clinical Practice Guidelines in the Netherlands: a prospect for continuous quality improvement in Physical Therapy (2003) Bekkering et al. A CDROM available from the Royal Dutch Society for Physical Therapy.[215]

Reviewing and piloting these guidelines

The GDG compiled a list of specialists, researchers and practitioners at all levels. They looked to their own departments and beyond to find reviewers who could read the guidelines and assess the practicality of their contents. Time constraints did not allow for piloting beyond this theoretical process. Table 12.1 includes a list of reviewers, their post and speciality at the time of the review.

The draft guidelines and a reviewers' comments sheet (Appendix I), were distributed to the reviewers on 4th May 2004. Comments returned were collated and discussed at the GDG meeting of 3rd June 2004. Many amendments were made; some examples are indicated below. Overall the advice given by the reviewers was extremely constructive and invaluable in assisting the GDG in producing this high quality document.

Table 12.1	Reviewers of this document	
Name	Post	Specialty
Joanna Birch	Clinical co-ordinator physiotherapy	Musculoskeletal physiotherapy
Annette Bishop	Research physiotherapist	Musculoskeletal physiotherapy
Julie Burge	Senior I physiotherapist	Musculoskeletal physiotherapy
Guy Canby	Lecturer/practitioner	Musculoskeletal physiotherapy
Ben Davies	Senior II physiotherapist	Musculoskeletal physiotherapy
Linda Exelby	Specialist physiotherapist	Musculoskeletal physiotherapy
Emma Fanning	Junior physiotherapist	General rotational post
Helen Gidlow	Spinal clinical specialist	Musculoskeletal physiotherapy
Mandy Grocutt	Accident and emergency consultant	Accident and emergency medicine
Penny Harber	Extended scope physiotherapist	Musculoskeletal A&E
Rachael Heyes	Senior II physiotherapist	Musculoskeletal – out-patients
Susan Hintze	Physiotherapy manager	Unstated
Tom Hughes	Senior II physiotherapist	Musculoskeletal physiotherapy
Michael Lee	Senior II physiotherapist	Musculoskeletal physiotherapy
Jeremy Lewis	Research physiotherapist	Musculoskeletal physiotherapy research
Fiona Ottewell	Head of physiotherapy	Musculoskeletal physiotherapy
Colette Owen	Senior I physiotherapist	Musculoskeletal physiotherapy
Helen Payne	Extended scope physiotherapist	A&E
Nicola Petty	Principal lecturer	Musculoskeletal physiotherapy
Patsy Rochester	Senior university lecturer	Musculoskeletal physiotherapy
Alison Sharp	Clinical specialist	Spinal & musculoskeletal physiotherapy
Toby Smith	Extended scope physiotherapist	Musculoskeletal physiotherapy
Joanne Stott	Senior I physiotherapist	Musculoskeletal – out-patients
Emma Thompson	Senior II physiotherapist	Rotational post
Janet Wakefield	Senior I physiotherapist	Musculoskeletal physiotherapy

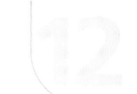

Examples of amendments made following review:

- A list of references in alphabetical order of author name was added (Appendix M) to enable the reader to readily access papers

- Minor adjustments were made to the writing style in the systematic review section

- The list of red flags was amended to include 'other conditions associated with instability or hypermobility' (section 3.6.4.3)

- The section on assessment was modified so that it did not assume a Maitland approach (section 3.6.5.2)

- The yellow flag section was adjusted to include post-traumatic stress reaction (section 3.4.4.6)

- Papers identified by reviewers that had not been included were obtained and considered for inclusion. Some were added e.g.[77,113–115] These were related to sections where a comprehensive search had not been conducted

- Numerous typing errors were corrected and some points tightened or clarified

- The accident and emergency consultant advised that those with serious pathology need immediate referral to the accident and emergency department; this was emphasised in the document (section 3.6.4.1).

Procedure for updating these guidelines

The systematic review and Delphi consensus methods will be updated in 2010.

At that time, consideration will be given to putting the Delphi questionnaire on the CSP website so that a wide range of member opinions can contribute to the 2010 edition of the guidelines. The Delphi technique is new within health care but potentially powerful in capturing expert opinion for guidelines production.

References

1   Hammond, R and Mead, J (2003). *Identifying national priorities for physical therapy clinical guideline development*. In: Abstracts from 14th International WCPT Congress, Barcelona, Spain, 7–12 June 2003. World confederation for Physical Thereapy, 2003, London

2   Spitzer, WO, Skovron, ML, Salmi, LR, Cassidy, JD, Duranceau, J, Suissa, S, Zeiss, E, Weinstein, JN and Nogbuk, N (1995). Scientific monograph of the Quebec Task Force on whiplash-associated disorders: Redefining 'Whiplash' and its management. *Spine* **20** (8)

3   Burton, K (2003). *Treatment guidelines: Is there a need?* In: Proceeding of Whiplash 2003 conference, Bath, England, 6–8 May 2003. Lyons Davidson Solicitors, 2003, Bristol

4   Mills, H and Horne, G (1986). Whiplash – manmade disease? *New Zealand Medical Journal* **99** (802), 373–374

5   Cote, P, Hogg-Johnson, S, Cassidy, JD, Carroll, L and Frank, JW (2001). The association between neck pain intensity, physical functioning, depressive symptomatology and time-to-claim-closure after whiplash. *Journal of Clinical Epidemiology* **54** (3), 275–286

6   Scholten-Peeters, GGM, Bekkering, GE, Verhagen, AP, van der Windt, DAW, Lanser, K, Hendriks, EJM and Oostendorp, RA (2002). Clinical practice guideline for the physiotherapy of patients with whiplash-associated disorders. *Spine* **27** (4), 412–422

7   Galasko, CS, Murray, PM, Pitcher, M, Chambers, H, Mansfield, S, Madden, M, Jordon, C, Kinsella, A and Hodson, M (1993). Neck sprains after road traffic accidents: a modern epidemic. *Injury* **24** (3), 155–157

8   Office for National Statistics (2002). *Road accident casualties: by road user type and severity 1992–2002: annual abstract of statistics*. Office for National Statistics. Available from: http://www.statistics.gov.uk/STATBASE/ssdataset.asp?vlnk=4031 (Accessed 6th May 2005)

9   Ferrari, R and Russell, AS (1999). Epidemiology of whiplash: an international dilemma. *Annals of the Rheumatic Diseases* **58** (1), 1–5

10   Field, MJ and Lohr, KNE (1992). *Guidelines for clinical practice: from development to use*. National Academy Press, Washington DC

11   Scottish Intercollegiate Guidelines Network (2001). *Sign 50: A guideline developers' handbook* Scottish Intercollegiate Guidelines Network. Available from: http://www.sign.ac.uk/guidelines/fulltext/50/index.html (Accessed on 3rd June 2005)

12   McClune, T, Burton, AK and Waddell, G (2002). Whiplash associated disorders: a review of the literature to guide patient information and advice. *Emergency Medical Journal* **19** (6), 499–506

13   Verhagen, AP, Peeters, GGM, de Bie, RA and Oostendorp, RA (2002). *Conservative treatment for whiplash*. The Cochrane Library: Update Software, Oxford

14   Binder, A (2002). Neck pain. *Clinical Evidence* (7), 1049–1062

15   Magee, DJ, Oborn-Barrett, E, Turner, S and Fenning, N (2000). A systematic overview of the effectiveness of physical therapy intervention on soft tissue neck injury following trauma. *Physiotherapy Canada* **52** (2), 111–130

16   Bogduk, N (2002). Manual therapy produces greater relief of neck pain than physiotherapy or general practitioner care. *Australian Journal of Physiotherapy* **48**, 240

17   Jull, G (2001). For self-perceived benefit from treatment for chronic neck pain, multimodal treatment is more effective than home exercises, and both are more effective than advice alone. *Australian Journal of Physiotherapy* **47** (3), 215

18   Kwan, O and Friel, J (2003). Management of chronic pain in whiplash injury. *Journal of Bone & Joint Surgery - British Volume* **85B** (6), 931–932

19   Meal, G (2002). A clinical trial investigating the possible effect of the supine cervical rotary manipulation and the supine rotary break manipulation in the treatment of mechanical neck pain: a pilot study. *Journal of Manipulative & Physiological Therapeutics* **25** (8), 541–542

20   Hoving, JL, Koes, B, de Vet, HC, van der Windt, DAW, Assendelft, WJ, Van Mameren, H, Deville, WLJM, Pool, JJM, Scholten, RJPM and Bouter, LM (2002). Manual therapy, physical therapy, or continued care by a general practitioner for patients with neck pain: A randomized controlled trial. *Annals of Internal Medicine* **136**, 713–722

21   Hurwitz, EL, Morgenstern, H, Harber, P, Kominski, GF, Yu, F and Adams, AH (2002). A randomized trial of chiropractic manipulation and mobilization for patients with neck pain: Clinical outcomes from the UCLA neck-pain study. *American Journal of Public Health* **92**, 1634–1641

22   Korthals-de Bos, IB, Hoving, JL, van Tulder, M, Rutten-van Molken, MP, Ader, HJ, de Vet, HC, Koes, B, Vondeling, H and Bouter, LM (2003). Cost effectiveness of physiotherapy, manual therapy, and general practitioner care for neck pain: economic evaluation alongside a randomised controlled trial. *British Medical Journal* **326** (7395), 911–914

23   Humphreys, BK and Irgens, PM (2002). The effect of a rehabilitation exercise program on head repositioning accuracy and reported levels of pain in chronic neck pain subjects. *Journal of Whiplash and Related Disorders* **1**, 99–112

24   Vendrig, AA, van Akkerveeken, PF and McWhorter, KR (2000). Results of a multimodal treatment program for patients with chronic symptoms after a whiplash injury of the neck. *Spine* **25** (2), 238–244

25   Wang, WT, Olson, SL, Campbell, AH, Hanten, WP and Gleeson, PB (2003). Effectiveness of physical therapy for patients with neck pain: an individualized approach using a clinical decision-making algorithm. *American Journal of Physical Medicine & Rehabilitation* **82** (3), 203–218

26   Scholten-Peeters, GGM, Verhagen, AP, Neeleman-van der Steen, CW, Hurkmans, JC, Wams, RW and Oostendorp, RA (2003). Randomized clinical trial of conservative treatment for patients with whiplash-associated disorders: considerations for the design and dynamic treatment protocol. *Journal of Manipulative & Physiological Therapeutics* **26** (7), 412–420

27   Evans, R, Bronfort, G, Nelson, B and Goldsmith, C (2002). Two-year follow-up of a randomized clinical trial of spinal manipulation and two types of exercise for patients with chronic neck pain. *Spine* **27**, 2383–2389

28   Kjellman, G and Oberg, B (2002). A randomized clinical trial comparing general exercise, McKenzie treatment and a control group in patients with neck pain. *Journal of Rehabilitation Medicine* **34** (4), 183–190

29   Rosenfeld, M, Seferiadis, A, Carlsson, J and Gunnarsson, R (2003). Active intervention in patients with whiplash-associated disorders improves long-term prognosis: a randomized controlled clinical trial. *Spine* **28** (22), 2491–2498

30   Thuile, C and Walzl, M (2002). Evaluation of electromagnetic fields in the treatment of pain in patients with lumbar radiculopathy or the whiplash syndrome. *Neurorehabilitation* **17**, 63–67

31   Wood, TG, Colloca, CJ and Matthews, R (2001). A pilot randomized clinical trial on the relative effect of instrumental (MFMA) versus manual (HVLA) manipulation in the treatment of cervical spine dysfunction. *Journal of Manipulative & Physiological Therapeutics* **24** (4), 260–271

32   Bonk, AD, Ferrari, R, Giebel, GD, Edelmann, M and Huser, R (2000). Prospective, randomized, controlled study of activity versus collar, and the natural history for whiplash injury, in Germany. World Congress on whiplash-associated disorders, Vancouver, British Columbia, Canada. February 1999. *Journal of Musculoskeletal Pain* **8** (1–2), 123–132

33   Borchgrevink, G, Kaasa, A, McDonagh, D, Stiles, TC, Haraldseth, O and Lereim, I (1998). Acute treatment of whiplash neck sprain injuries: a randomized trial of treatment during the first 14 days after a car accident. *Spine* **23** (1), 25–31

34   Fitz-Ritson, D (1995). Phasic exercises for cervical rehabilitation after "whiplash" trauma. *Journal of Manipulative and Physiological Therapeutics* **18** (1), 21–24

35   Foley-Nolan, D, Moore, K, Codd, M, Barry, C, O'Connor, P and Coughlan, RJ (1992). Low energy high frequency pulsed electromagnetic therapy for acute whiplash injuries. A double blind randomized controlled study. *Scandinavian Journal of Rehabilitation Medicine* **24** (1), 51–59

36   Gennis, P, Miller, L, Gallagher, EJ, Giglio, J, Carter, W and Nathanson, N (1996). The effect of soft cervical collars on persistent neck pain in patients with whiplash injury. *Academic Emergency Medicine* **3** (6), 568–573

37   Hendriks, O and Horgan, A (1996). Ultra-reiz current as an adjunct to standard physiotherapy treatment of the acute whiplash patient. *Physiotherapy Ireland* **17** (1), 3–7

38   McKinney, LA, Dornan, JO and Ryan, M (1989). The role of physiotherapy in the management of acute neck sprains following road-traffic accidents. *Archives of Emergency Medicine* **6** (1), 27–33

39   McKinney, LA (1989). Early mobilisation and outcome in acute sprains of the neck. *British Medical Journal* **299** (6706), 1006–1008

40   Mealy, K, Brennan, H and Fenelon, GC (1986). Early mobilization of acute whiplash injuries. *British Medical Journal (Clinical Research ed.)* **292** (6521), 656–657

41   Pennie, BH and Agambar, LJ (1990). Whiplash injuries. A trial of early management. *Journal of Bone & Joint Surgery – British Volume* **72** (2), 277–279

42   Provinciali, L, Baroni, M, Illuminati, L and Ceravolo, MG (1996). Multimodal treatment to prevent the late whiplash syndrome. *Scandinavian Journal of Rehabilitation Medicine* **28** (2), 105–111

43   Rosenfeld, M, Gunnarsson, R and Borenstein, P (2000). Early intervention in whiplash-associated disorders: a comparison of two treatment protocols. *Spine* **25** (14), 1782–1787

44   Soderlund, A, Olerud, C and Lindberg, P (2000). Acute whiplash-associated disorders (WAD): the effects of early mobilization and prognostic factors in long-term symptomatology. *Clinical Rehabilitation* **14** (5), 457–467

45   Centre for Evidence-Based Physiotherapy (1999). *The PEDro scale*. Centre for Evidence-Based Physiotherapy, Sydney. Available from: http://www.pedro.fhs.usyd.edu.au/scale_item.html (Accessed 2nd June 2005)

46   Verhagen, AP, de Vet, HC, de Bie, RA, Kessels, AG, Boers, M, Bouter, LM and Knipschild, PG (1998). The Delphi list: a criteria list for quality assessment of randomized clinical trials for conducting systematic reviews developed by Delphi consensus. *Journal of Clinical Epidemiology* **51** (12), 1235–1241

47   Maher, CG, Sherrington, C, Herbert, RD, Moseley, AM and Elkins, M (2003). Reliability of the PEDro Scale for rating quality of randomized controlled trials. *Physical Therapy* **83** (8), 713–721

48   Chartered Society of Physiotherapy (2003). *Guidance for developing clinical guidelines*. The Chartered Society of Physiotherapy, London. Available from: http://www.csp.org.uk/libraryandinformation/publications/view.cfm?id=275 (Accessed 6th May 2005)

49   Murphy, MK, Black, NA, Lamping, DL, McKee, CM, Sanderson, CFB, Ashkam, J and Marteau, T (1998). Consensus development methods and their use in clinical guideline development. In *Health Technologies Assessment*; **2** (3). Available from http://www.mrw.interscience.wiley.com/cochrane/clhta/articles/HTA-988414/frame.html (Accessed 2nd June 2005)

50   Alder, M and Ziglio, E (1996). *Gazing into the oracle. The Delphi method and its application to social policy and public health*. Jessica Kingsley, London.

51   Pope, C and Mays, N (1999). *Qualitative research in health care*. 2nd Edition. BMJ books, London.

52   Sackman, H (1975). *Delphi critique*. Lexington Books, Lexington MA.

53   McKenna, HP (1994). The Delphi technique: a worthwhile research approach for nursing? *Journal of Advanced Nursing* **19** (6), 1221–1225

54   Boyce, W, Gowland, C, Russell, D, Goldsmith, C, Rosenbaum, P, Plews, N and Lane, M (1993). Consensus methodology in the development and content validation of a gross motor performance measure. *Physiotherapy Canada* **45** (2), 94–100

55   Bramwell, L and Hykawy, E (1999). The Delphi Technique: a possible tool for predicting future events in nursing education. *Canadian Journal of Nursing Research* **30** (4), 47–58

56 AGREE Collaboration (2001). *AGREE Instrument: Appraisal of guidelines for research and evaluation*. The AGREE Collaboration. Available from: http://www.agreecollaboration.org (accessed on 6th May 2005)

57 Crowe, H (1928). *Injuries to the cervical spine*. In Annual meeting of Western Orthopaedic Association, San Francisco, California

58 Eck, JC, Hodges, SD and Humphreys, SC (2001). Whiplash: a review of a commonly misunderstood injury. *American Journal of Medicine* **110** (8), 651–656

59 Panjabi, MM, Cholewicki, J, Nibu, K, Grauer, JN, Babat, LB and Dvorak, J (1998). Mechanism of whiplash injury. *Clinical Biomechanics* **13** (4–5), 239–249

60 Walz, FH and Muser, MH (2000). Biomechanical assessment of soft tissue cervical spine disorders and expert opinion in low speed collisions. *Accident Analysis and Prevention* **32** (2), 161–165

61 Bogduk, N and Yoganandan, N (2001). Biomechanics of the cervical spine Part 3: minor injuries. *Clinical Biomechanics* **16** (4), 267–275

62 Panjabi, MM, Pearson, AM, Ito, S, Ivancic, PC and Wang, JL (2004). Cervical spine curvature during simulated whiplash. *Clinical Biomechanics* **19** (1), 1–9

63 Tenenbaum, A, Rivano Fischer, M, Tjell, C, Edblom, M and Sunnerhagen, KS (2002). The Quebec classification and a new Swedish classification for whiplash-associated disorders in relation to life satisfaction in patients at high risk of chronic functional impairment and disability. *Journal of Rehabilitation Medicine* **34** (3), 114–118

64 Hartling, L, Brison, RJ, Ardern, C and Pickett, W (2001). Prognostic value of the Quebec classification of whiplash-associated disorders. *Spine* **26** (1), 36–41

65 Centeno, C (2003). *Whiplash prognosis*. In: Proceedings of 2003 Whiplash conference, Bath, England. 6–8 May 2003. Lyons Davidson Solicitors, 2003, Bristol

66 Hammacher, ER and van der Werken, C (1996). Acute neck sprain: 'whiplash' reappraised. *Injury* **27** (7), 463–466

67 Karlsborg, M, Smed, A, Jespersen, H, Stephensen, S, Cortsen, M, Jennum, P, Herning, M, Korfitsen, E and Werdelin, L (1997). A prospective study of 39 patients with whiplash injury. *Acta Neurologica Scandinavica* **95** (2), 65–72

68 Galasko, CS, Murray, PA and Pitcher, M (2000). Prevalence and long-term disability following whiplash-associated disorder. World Congress on whiplash-associated disorders, Vancouver, British Columbia, Canada. February 1999. *Journal of Musculoskeletal Pain* **8** (1–2), 15–27

69 Bogduk, N (1999). The neck. *Baillieres Best Practice and Research in Clinical Rheumatology* **13** (2), 261–285

70 Soderlund, A and Lindberg, P (1999). Long-term functional and psychological problems in whiplash associated disorders. *International Journal of Rehabilitation Research* **22** (2), 77–84

71 Sullivan, MJ, Hall, E, Bartolacci, R, Sullivan, ME and Adams, H (2002). Perceived cognitive deficits, emotional distress and disability following whiplash injury. *Pain Research & Management* **7** (3), 120–126

72 Squires, B, Gargan, MF and Bannister, GC (1996). Soft-tissue injuries of the cervical spine. 15-year follow-up. *Journal of Bone & Joint Surgery – British Volume* **78** (6), 955–957

73 Suissa, S, Harder, S and Veilleux, M (2001). The relation between initial symptoms and signs and the prognosis of whiplash. *European Spine Journal* **10** (1), 44–49

74 Mulhall, KJ, Moloney, M, Burke, TE and Masterson, E (2003). Chronic neck pain following road traffic accidents in an Irish setting and it's relationship to seat belt use and low back pain. *Irish Medical Journal* **96** (2), 53–54

75 Otremski, I, Marsh, JL, McLardy-Smith, PD and Newman, RJ (1989). Soft tissue cervical spinal injuries in motor vehicle accidents. *Injury* **20** (6), 349–351

76 Schuller, E, Eisenmenger, W and Beier, G (2000). Whiplash injury in low speed car accidents: assessment of biomechanical cervical spine loading and injury prevention in a forensic sample. World Congress on whiplash-associated disorders in Vancouver, British Columbia, Canada. February 1999. *Journal of Musculoskeletal Pain* **8** (1–2), 55–67

77   Scholten-Peeters, GG, Verhagen, AP, Bekkering, GE, van der Windt, DA, Barnsley, L, Oostendorp, RA and Hendriks, EJ (2003). Prognostic factors of whiplash-associated disorders: a systematic review of prospective cohort studies. *Pain* **104** (1-2), 303–322

78   Waddell, G, Burton, AK and McClune, T (2001). *The whiplash book*. The Stationery Office, Norwich.

79   Jakobsson, L, Lundell, B, Norin, H and Isaksson Hellman, I (2000). WHIPS – Volvo's whiplash protection study. *Accident Analysis and Prevention* **32** (2), 307–319

80   Dolinis, J (1997). Risk factors for 'whiplash' in drivers: a cohort study of rear-end traffic crashes. *Injury* **28** (3), 173–179

81   Salmi, LR, Thomas, H, Fabry, JJ and Girard, R (1989). The effect of the 1979 French seatbelt law on the nature and severity of injuries to front seat occupants. *Accident Analysis and Prevention* **21**, 589–594

82   Barancik, JI, Kramer, CF and Thode, HC (1989). *Epidemiology of motor vehicle injuries in Suffolk County, New York before and after enactment of the New York State seat belt use law.* US Department of Transportation, National Highway Traffic Safety Administration, Washington DC

83   Tunbridge, RJ (1990). The long term effect of seat belt legislation on road user injury patterns. *Health Bulletin (Edinburgh)* **48** (6), 347–349

84   Bourbeau, R, Desjardins, D, Maag, U and Laberge-Nadeau, C (1993). Neck injuries among belted and unbelted occupants of the front seat of cars. *Journal of Trauma* **35** (5), 794–799

85   Versteegen, GJ, Kingma, J, Meijler, WJ and ten Duis, HJ (2000). Neck sprain after motor vehicle accidents in drivers and passengers. *European Spine Journal* **9** (6), 547–552

86   Sterner, Y, Toolanen, G, Gerdle, B and Hildingsson, C (2003). The incidence of whiplash trauma and the effects of different factors on recovery. *Journal of Spinal Disorders & Techniques* **16** (2), 195–199

87   Croft, PR, Lewis, M, Papageorgiou, AC, Thomas, E, Jayson, MI, Macfarlane, GJ and Silman, AJ (2001). Risk factors for neck pain: a longitudinal study in the general population. *Pain* **93** (3), 317–325

88   Schrader, H, Obelieniene, D, Bovim, G, Surkiene, D, Mickeviciene, D, Miseviciene, I and Sand, T (1996). Natural evolution of late whiplash syndrome outside the medicolegal context. *Lancet* **347** (9010), 1207–1211

89   Harder, S, Veilleux, M and Suissa, S (1998). The effect of socio-demographic and crash-related factors on the prognosis of whiplash. *Journal of Clinical Epidemiology* **51** (5), 377–384

90   McLean, AJ (1995). Neck injury severity and vehicle design. In: Griffiths M, Brown J (eds) *Biomechanics of neck injury.* Proceedings of a seminar held in Adelaide, Australia pp.47–50. NH&MRC Road Accident Research Unit, University of Adelaide. Institution of Engineers, Canberra

91   Versteegen, GJ, Kingma, J, Meijler, WJ and ten Duis, HJ (1998). Neck sprain in patients injured in car accidents: a retrospective study covering the period 1970–1994. *European Spine Journal* **7** (3), 195–200

92   Ryan, GA (2000). Etiology and outcomes of whiplash: review and update. World Congress on whiplash-associated disorders in Vancouver, British Columbia, Canada. February 1999. *Journal of Musculoskeletal Pain* **8** (1–2), 3–14

93   Bring, G, Bjornstig, U and Westman, G (1996). Gender patterns in minor head and neck injuries: an analysis of casualty register data. *Accident Analysis and Prevention* **28** (3), 359–369

94   Chapline, JF, Ferguson, SA, Lillis, RP, Lund, AK and Williams, AF (2000). Neck pain and head restraint position relative to the driver's head in rear-end collisions. *Accident Analysis and Prevention* **32** (2), 287–297

95   Waddell, G and Main, CJ (1984). Assessment of severity in low-back disorders. *Spine* **9** (2), 204–208

96   Main, CJ and Watson, PJ (1999). Psychological aspects of pain. *Manual Therapy* **4** (4), 203–215

97 Watson, PJ (1999). Psychosocial assessment: the emergence of a new fashion, or a new tool in physiotherapy for musculoskeletal pain? *Physiotherapy* **85** (10), 533–535

98 Symonds, TL, Burton, AK, Tillotson, KM and Main, CJ (1996). Do attitudes and beliefs influence work loss due to low back trouble? *Occupational Medicine* **46** (1), 25–32

99 Waddell, G and Burton, AK (2001). Occupational health guidelines for the management of low back pain at work: evidence review. *Occupational Medicine* **51** (2), 124–135

100 Grossi, G, Soares, JJ, Angesleva, J and Perski, A (1999). Psychosocial correlates of long-term sick-leave among patients with musculoskeletal pain. *Pain* **80** (3), 607–619

101 Kendall, NAS, Linton, SJ and Main, CJ (1997). *Guide to assessing psychological yellow flags in acute low back pain: risk factors for long term disability and work loss.* Accident Rehabilitation & Compensation Insursance Corporation of New Zealand and the National Health Committee, Wellington

102 Waddell, G (1998). *The Back Pain Revolution*. Churchill Livingstone, Edinburgh

103 Schofferman, J and Wasserman, S (1994). Successful treatment of low back pain and neck pain after a motor vehicle accident despite litigation. *Spine* **19** (9), 1007–1010

104 Maimaris, C, Barnes, MR and Allen, MJ (1988). 'Whiplash injuries' of the neck: a retrospective study. *Injury* **19** (6), 393–396

105 Parmar, HV and Raymakers, R (1993). Neck injuries from rear impact road traffic accidents: prognosis in persons seeking compensation. *Injury* **24** (2), 75–78

106 Cote, P, Cassidy, JD, Carroll, L, Frank, JW and Bombardier, C (2001). A systematic review of the prognosis of acute whiplash and a new conceptual framework to synthesize the literature. *Spine* **26** (19), E445–458

107 Sterling, M, Kenardy, J, Jull, G and Vicenzino, B (2003). The development of psychological changes following whiplash injury. *Pain* **106** (3), 481–489

108 Main, CJ and Burton, AK (2000). Economic and occupational influences on pain and disability. In Main, CJ and Spanswick, CS, eds., *Pain management – An interdisciplinary approach pp63–87.* Churchill Livingstone, London

109 Brison, RJ, Hartling, L and Pickett, W (2000). A prospective study of acceleration-extension injuries following rear-end motor vehicle collisions. World Congress on whiplash-associated disorders, Vancouver, British Columbia, Canada. February 1999. *Journal of Musculoskeletal Pain* **8** (1–2), 97–113

110 Mayou, R and Radanov, BP (1996). Whiplash neck injury. *Journal of Psychosomatic Research* **40** (5), 461–474

111 Bogduk, N and Lord, S (1998). Cervical spine disorders. *Current Opinion in Rheumatology* **10** (2), 110–115

112 Lord, S, Barnsley, L, Wallis, BJ and Bogduk, N (1996). Chronic cervical zygapophysial joint pain after whiplash: a placebo-controlled prevalence study. *Spine* **21** (15), 1737–1745

113 Koelbaek Johansen, M, Graven-Nielsen, T, Schou Olesen, A and Arendt-Nielsen, L (1999). Generalised muscular hyperalgesia in chronic whiplash syndrome. *Pain* **83** (2), 229–234

114 Banic, B, Petersen-Felix, S, Andersen, OK, Radanov, BP, Villiger, PM, Arendt Nielsen, L and Curatolo, M (2004). Evidence for spinal cord hypersensitivity in chronic pain after whiplash injury and in fibromyalgia. *Pain* **107** (1–2), 7–15

115 Curatolo, M, Petersen-Felix, S, Arendt-Nielsen, L, Giani, C, Zbinden, AM and Radanov, BP (2001). Central hypersensitivity in chronic pain after whiplash injury. *Clinical Journal of Pain* **17** (4), 306–315

116 Amundson, GM (1994). The evaluation and treatment of cervical whiplash. *Current Opinion in Orthopedics* **5** (2), 17–27

117 Schrader, H, Obelieniene, D and Ferrari, R (2000). Temporomandibular and whiplash injury in Lithuania. World Congress on whiplash-associated disorders, Vancouver, British Columbia, Canada. February 1999. *Journal of Musculoskeletal Pain* **8** (1–2), 133–142

118 Bodguk, N (1986). The anatomy and pathophysiology of whiplash. *Clinical Biomechanics* **1** (2), 92–101

119 Barnsley, L, Lord, S and Bogduk, N (1994). Whiplash injury. *Pain* **58** (3), 283–307

120 Heikkila, HV and Wenngren, BI (1998). Cervicocephalic kinesthetic sensibility, active range of cervical motion, and oculomotor function in patients with whiplash injury. *Archives of Physical Medicine & Rehabilitation* **79** (9), 1089–1094

121 Schmand, B, Lindeboom, J, Schagen, S, Heijt, R, Koene, T and Hamburger, HL (1998). Cognitive complaints in patients after whiplash injury: the impact of malingering. *Journal of Neurology, Neurosurgery, and Psychiatry* **64** (3), 339–343

122 Department of Health (2001). *Department of Health Guide: Reference guide to consent for examination or treatment.* Department of Health, London. Available from: www.dh.gov.uk/PublicationsAndStatistics/Publications/PublicationsPolicyAndGuidance/Publications PolicyAndGuidanceArticle/fs/en?CONTENT_ID=4006757&chk=snmdw8 (Accessed 6th May 2005)

123 Chartered Society of Physiotherapy (2005). *Core Standards.* The Chartered Society of Physiotherapy, London

124 Royal College of General Practitioners (1999). *Clinical guidelines for the management of acute low back pain.* Royal College of General Practitioners, London

125 Clinical Standards Advisory Group (CSAG) (1994). *Back pain.* HMSO, London

126 Magee, DJ (1997). *Orthopaedic Physical Assessment.* Saunders, New York

127 Boyling, JD and Palastanga, N (1998). *Grieve's modern manual therapy.* Churchill Livingstone, London

128 Petty, N and Moore, A (2001). *A neuromusculoskeletal examination and assessment: a handbook for therapists.* Churchill Livingstone, Edinburgh

129 Maitland, GD, Hengeveld, E and Banks, K (2001). *Maitland's vertebral manipulation.* Butterworth Heinmann, Oxford

130 Dall'Alba, PT, Sterling, MM, Treleaven, JM, Edwards, SL and Jull, G (2001). Cervical range of motion discriminates between asymptomatic persons and those with whiplash. *Spine* **26** (19), 2090–2094

131 Yeung, E, Jones, M and Hall, B (1997). The response to the slump test in a group of female whiplash patients. *Australian Journal of Physiotherapy* **43** (4), 245–252

132 Jull, G (2000). Deep cervical flexor muscle dysfunction in whiplash. World Congress on whiplash-associated disorders, Vancouver, British Columbia, Canada. February 1999. *Journal of Musculoskeletal Pain* **8** (1–2), 143–154

133 Loudon, JK, Ruhl, M and Field, E (1997). Ability to reproduce head position after whiplash injury. *Spine* **22** (8), 865–868

134 Barker, S, Kesson, M, Ashmore, J, Turner, G, Conway, J and Stevens, D (2000). Guidance for pre-manipulative testing of the cervical spine. *Manual Therapy* **5** (1), 37–40

135 RCR Working Party (2003). *Making the best use of a department of clinical radiology: guidelines for doctors, (5th edition).* The Royal College of Radiologists, London.

136 Matsumoto, M, Fujimura, Y, Suzuki, N, Toyama, Y and Shiga, H (1998). Cervical curvature in acute whiplash injuries: prospective comparative study with asymptomatic subjects. *Injury* **29** (10), 775–778

137 Borchgrevink, G, Smevik, O, Haave, I, Haraldseth, O, Nordby, A and Lereim, I (1997). MRI of cerebrum and cervical columna within two days after whiplash neck sprain injury. *Injury* **28** (5–6), 331–335

138 Gotzsche, PC (2002). Non-steroidal anti-inflammatory drugs. *Clinical Evidence* (7), 1063–1070

139 PRODIGY (2001). *Prodigy Clinical Guidance – Neck Pain.* Department of Health, London. Available from: http://www.prodigy.nhs.uk/guidance.asp?gt=Neck%20pain (Accessed on 6th May 2005)

140 Gross, AR, Kay, TM, Kennedy, C, Gasner, D, Hurley, L, Yardley, K, Hendry, L and McLaughlin, L (2002a). Clinical practice guideline on the use of manipulation or mobilization in the treatment of adults with mechanical neck disorders. *Manual Therapy* 7 (4), 193–205

141 Kjellman, G, Skargren, EI and Oberg, BE (1999). A critical analysis of randomised clinical trials on neck pain and treatment efficacy. A review of the literature. *Scandinavian Journal of Rehabilitation Medicine* 31 (3), 139–152

142 Dabbs, V and Lauretti, WJ (1995). A risk assessment of cervical manipulation vs. NSAIDs for the treatment of neck pain. *Journal of Manipulative and Physiological Therapeutics* 18 (8), 530–536

143 Stevinson, C and Ernst, E (2002). Risks associated with spinal manipulation. *American Journal of Medicine* 112 (7), 566–571

144 Sarig-Bahat, H (2003). Evidence for exercise therapy in mechanical neck disorders. *Manual Therapy* 8 (1), 10–20

145 Karjalainen, K, Malmivaara, A, van Tulder, M, Roine, R, Jauhiainen, M, Hurri, H and Koes, B (2003). *Multidisciplinary biopsychosocial rehabilitation for subacute low back pain among working age adults.* The Cochrane Library, Update Software, Oxford

146 White, AR and Ernst, E (1999). A systematic review of randomized controlled trials of acupuncture for neck pain. *Rheumatology* 38 (2), 143–147

147 Gross, AR, Aker, PD, Goldsmith, C and Peloso, P (2002b). *Patient education for mechanical neck disorders.* The Cochrane Library, Update Software, Oxford

148 van der Heijden, GJ, Beurskens, AJ, Koes, B, Assendelft, WJ, de Vet, HC and Bouter, LM (1995). The efficacy of traction for back and neck pain: a systematic, blinded review of randomized clinical trial methods. *Physical Therapy* 75 (2), 93–104

149 Gross, AR, Aker, PD, Goldsmith, C and Peloso, P (2002c). *Physical medicine modalities for mechanical neck disorders.* The Cochrane Library, Update Software, Oxford

150 Albright, J, Allman, R, Bonfiglio, RP, Conill, A, Dobkin, B, Guccione, AA, Hasson, SM, Russo, R, Shekelle, P, Susman, JL, Brosseau, L, Tugwell, P, Wells, GA, Robinson, VA, Graham, ID, Shea, BJ, McGowan, J, Peterson, J, Poulin, L, Tousignant, M, Corriveau, H, Morin, M, Pelland, L, Laferriere, L, Casimiro, L and Tremblay, LE (2001). Philadelphia panel evidence-based clinical practice guidelines on selected rehabilitation interventions for neck pain. *Physical Therapy* 81 (10), 1701–1717

151 Bronfort, G, Evans, R, Nelson, B, Aker, PD, Goldsmith, C and Vernon, H (2001). A randomized clinical trial of exercise and spinal manipulation for patients with chronic neck pain. *Spine* 26 (7), 788–797

152 Mior, S (2001). Manipulation and mobilization in the treatment of chronic pain. *Clinical Journal of Pain* 17 (4), Supplement: S70–76

153 Smith, LA, Oldman, AD, McQuay, HJ and Moore, RA (2000). Teasing apart quality and validity in systematic reviews: an example from acupuncture trials in chronic neck and back pain. *Pain* 86 (1–2), 119–132

154 Irnich, D, Behrens, N, Molzen, H, Konig, A, Gleditsch, J, Krauss, M, Natalis, M, Senn, E, Beyer, A and Schops, P (2001). Randomised trial of acupuncture compared with conventional massage and "sham" laser acupuncture for treatment of chronic neck pain. *British Medical Journal* 322 (7302), 1574–1578

155 Karjalainen, K, Malmivaara, A, van Tulder, M, Roine, R, Jauhiainen, M, Hurri, H and Koes, B (2003b). *Multidisciplinary biopsychosocial rehabilitation for neck and shoulder pain among working age adults* The Cochrane Library: Update Software, Oxford

156 Department of Health (2000). *The NHS Plan.* Department of Health, London

157   Chartered Society of Physiotherapy (2002). *Rules of professional conduct*. Chartered Society of Physiotherapy, London

158   Health Professions Council (2003). *Standards of proficiency – physiotherapists*. Health Professions Council, London

159   Barr, J and Threlkeld, AJ (2000). Patient-practitioner collaboration in clinical decision-making. *Physiotherapy Research International* **5** (4), 254–260

160   Stewart, M and Roter, D (1989). *Communicating with medical patients*. Sage Publications, New York

161   Ewles, L and Simnett, I (1992). *Promoting health a practical guide*. Scutari Press, London

162   Jensen, GM and Lorish, CD (1994). Promoting patient cooperation with exercise programs: linking research, theory, and practice. A*rthritis Care and Research* **7** (4), 181–189

163   Brody, DS, Miller, SM, Lerman, CE, Smith, DG and Caputo, GC (1989). Patient perception of involvement in medical care: relationship to illness attitudes and outcomes. *Journal of General Internal Medicine* **4** (6), 506–511

164   Baker, SM, Marshak, HH, Rice, GT and Zimmerman, GJ (2001). Patient participation in physical therapy goal setting. *Physical Therapy* **81** (5), 1118–1126

165   Richardson, K and Moran, S (1995). Developing standards for patient information. *International Journal of Health Care Quality Assurance* **8** (7), 27–31

166   Moore, A and Jull, G (2001). The art of listening. *Manual Therapy* **6** (3)

167   Knowles, M (1983). The modern practice of adult education from pedagogy to androgogy. In: Tight, MM, ed., *Adult Learning and Education, pp.*53–70. Croom Helm in association with the Open University, London

168   Moore, A, Hilton, R, Morris, J, Calladine, L and Bristow, H (1997). *The clinical educator – role development*. Churchill Livingstone, Edinburgh

169   Honey, P and Mumford, A (1986). *The manual of learning styles*. Printique, London.

170   Rodwell, CM (1996). An analysis of the concept of empowerment. *Journal of Advanced Nursing* **23** (2), 305–313

171   Rollnick, S, Mason, P and Butler, C (1999). *Health behaviour changes, A guide for practitioners*. Churchill Livingstone, Edinburgh

172   Bandura, A and Walter, RH (1963). *Social learning and personality development*. Thinehart & Winston, New York

173   Pietrobon, R, Coeytaux, RR, Carey, TS, Richardson, WJ and DeVellis, RF (2002). Standard scales for measurement of functional outcome for cervical pain or dysfunction: a systematic review. *Spine* **27** (5), 515–522

174   Huijbregts, MP, Myers, AM, Kay, TM and Gavin, TS (2002). Systematic outcome measurement in clinical practice: challenges experienced by physiotherapists. *Physiotherapy Canada* **54** (1), 25–31, 36

175   Huskisson, EC (1974). Measurement of pain. *Lancet* **2** (7889), 1127–1131

176   Vernon, H and Mior, S (1991). The neck disability index: a study of reliability and validity. *Journal of Manipulative Physiological Therapeutics* **14** (7), 409-415

177   Vernon, H (1996). The neck disability index: patient assessment and outcome monitoring in whiplash. *Journal of Musculoskeletal Pain* **4** (4), 95–104

178   Stratford, PW, Riddle, DL, Binkley, JM, Spadoni, G, Westaway, MD and Padfield, B (1999). Using the Neck Disability Index to make decisions concerning individual patients. *Physiotherapy Canada* **51** (2), 107–112

179   Vernon, H (2000). Assessment of self-rated disability, impairment, and sincerity of effort in whiplash-associated disorder. *Journal of Musculoskeletal Pain* **8**, 1–2

180 Westaway, MD, Stratford, PW and Binkley, JM (1998). The patient-specific functional scale: validation of its use in persons with neck dysfunction. *Journal of Orthopaedic and Sports Physical Therapy* **27** (5), 331–338

181 Paterson, C (1996). Measuring outcomes in primary care: a patient generated measure, MYMOP, compared with the SF-36 health survey. *British Medical Journal* **312** (7037), 1016–1020

182 Vlaeyen, J, Kole-Snijders, A, Boern, R, van Eek, H (1995). Fear of movement / (re)injury in chronic low back pain and its relation to behavioural performance. *Pain* **62**, 363–372

183 Crombez, G, Vlaeyen, JW, Heuts, PH and Lysens, R (1999). Pain-related fear is more disabling than pain itself: evidence on the role of pain-related fear in chronic back pain disability. *Pain* **80** (1-2), 329–339

184 Swinkels-Meewisse, EJ, Swinkels, RA, Verbeek, AL, Vlaeyen, JW and Oostendorp, RA (2003). Psychometric properties of the Tampa Scale for kinesiophobia and the fear-avoidance beliefs questionnaire in acute low back pain. *Manual Therapy* **8** (1), 29–36

185 Woby, SR, Roach, NK, Watson, PJ, Birch, KM and Urmston, M (2002). A further analysis of the psychometric properties of the Tampa Scale for Kinesiophobia (TSK). *Journal of Bone & Joint Surgery – British Volume* **84-B** (Supp III) (49)

186 Woby, SR, Watson, PJ, Roach, NK and Urmston, M (2003). *Psychometric properties of the Tampa scale for kinesiophobia*. Poster in 4th Congress of The European Federation of the International Association for the Study of Pain Chapters (Pain in Europe IV), Prague, Czech Republic. September 2003

187 Chartered Society of Physiotherapy (2000). *Clinical audit tools*. The Chartered Society of Physiotherapy, London

188 Zigmond, AS and Snaith, RP (1983). The hospital anxiety and depression scale. *Acta Psychiatrica Scandinavica* **67** (6), 361–370

189 Herrmann, C (1997). International experiences with the hospital anxiety and depression scale – a review of validation data and clinical results. *Journal of Psychosomatic Research* **42** (1), 17–41

190 Aylard, PR, Gooding, JH, McKenna, PJ and Snaith, RP (1987). A validation study of three anxiety and depression self-assessment scales. *Journal of Psychosomatic Research* **31** (2), 261–268

191 Greenough, CG and Fraser, RD (1991). Comparison of eight psychometric instruments in unselected patients with back pain. *Spine* **16** (9), 1068–1074

192 Upadhyaya, AK and Stanley, I (1993). Hospital anxiety depression scale. *British Journal of General Practice* **43** (373), 349–350

193 Anderson, KO, Dowds, BN, Pelletz, RE, Edwards, WT and Peeters-Asdourian, C (1995). Development and initial validation of a scale to measure self-efficacy beliefs in patients with chronic pain. *Pain* **63** (1), 77–84

194 Chartered Society of Physiotherapy (2000). *Reports for legal purposes: Information paper number PA1*. The Chartered Society of Physiotherapy, London

195 Bekkering, GE (2004). *Physiotherapy guidelines for low back pain: development, implementation and evaluation, (PhD thesis.)* Dutch Institute of Allied Health Care and the Institute for Research in Extramural Medicine (EMGO Institute) of the VU University Medical Centre

196 Haines, A and Donald, A (1998). *Getting research findings into practice*. BMJ Books, London

197 Feder, G, Eccles, M, Grol, R, Griffiths, C and Grimshaw, J (1999). Clinical guidelines: using clinical guidelines. *British Medical Journal* **318** (7185), 728–730

198 Feder, G (1994). Management of mild hypertension: which guidelines to follow? *British Medical Journal* **308**, 470–471

199 Grimshaw, J (2001). Changing provider behaviour: an overview of systematic reviews of interventions. *Medical Care* **39** (8)

200 Foster, NE and Doughty, GM (2003). *Dissemination and implementation of back pain guidelines: perspectives of musculoskeletal physiotherapists and managers.* Poster presentation in 6th International forum for low back pain research in primary care. Linkping, Sweden. May 2003

201 Doughty, GM and Foster, NE (2003). *Overcoming dissemination and implementation barriers to using clinical practice guidelines in physiotherapy.* Poster presentation in Defining practice, The Chartered Society of Physiotherapy annual Congess 17th–19th October 2003. Birmingham, UK

202 Mondloch, MV, Cole, DC and Frank, JW (2001). Does how you do depend on how you think you'll do? A systematic review of the evidence for a relation between patients' recovery expectations and health outcomes. *Canadian Medical Association Journal* **165** (2), 174–179

203 Thomas, E, Croft, PR, Paterson, SM, Dziedzic, K and Hay, EM (2004). What influences participants' treatment preference and can it influence outcome? Results from a primary care-based randomised trial for shoulder pain. *British Journal of General Practice* **54** (499), 93–96

204 van Tulder, M, Kovacs, F, Muller, G, Airaksinen, O, Balague, F, Broos, L, Burton, K, Gil del Real, MT, Hanninen, O, Henrotin, Y, Hildebrandt, J, Indahl, A, Leclerc, A, Manniche, C, Tilscher, H, Ursin, H, Vleeming, A and Zanoli, G (2002). European guidelines for the management of low back pain. *Acta Orthopaedica Scandinavica* **73** (305), 20–25

205 Rousseau, N, McColl, E, Newton, J, Grimshaw, J and Eccles, M (2003). Practice based, longitudinal, qualitative interview study of computerised evidence based guidelines in primary care. *British Medical Journal* **326** (7384), 314

206 Eccles, M, McColl, E, Steen, N, Rousseau, N, Grimshaw, J, Parkin, D and Purves, I (2002). Effect of computerised evidence based guidelines on management of asthma and angina in adults in primary care: cluster randomised controlled trial. *British Medical Journal* **325** (7370), 941

207 Evans, DW, Foster, NE, Vogel, S and Breen, AC (2003). *Implementing evidence-based practice in the UK physical therapy professions: Do they want it and do they need it?* Poster presentation at 6th International forum for low back pain research in primary care. Linkping, Sweden. May 2003

208 Freemantle, N, Harvey, E, Grimshaw, J, Wolf, F, Bero, L and Grilli, R (1996). *The effectiveness of printed educational materials in changing the behaviour of health care professionals.* The Cochrane Library, Update Software, Oxford.

209 Bero, L, Grilli, R, Grimshaw, J and Oxman, AD (1998). *The Cochrane effective practice and organisation of care review group.* The Cochrane Library, Update Software, Oxford.

210 Wensing, M, van der Weijden, T and Grol, R (1998). Implementing guidelines and innovations in general practice: which interventions are effective? *British Journal of General Practice* **48** (427), 991–997

211 Bekkering, GE, Engers, AJ, Wensing, M, Hendriks, HJ, van Tulder, M, Oostendorp, RA and Bouter, LM (2003). Development of an implementation strategy for physiotherapy guidelines on low back pain. *Australian Journal of Physiotherapy* **49** (3), 208–214

212 Grol, R and Jones, R (2000). Twenty years of implementation research. *Family Practice* **17** Suppl 1, 32–35

213 Motor Accidents Authority of New South Wales (2001). *Guidelines for the management of whiplash associated disorders.* Motor Accidents Authority of New South Wales. Available from: http://www.maa.nsw.gov.au/injury43whiplash.htm (Accesed on 6th May 2005)

214 Agencie Nationale d'Acreditation et d'Evaluation en Sante (2003). *Physiotherapy in common neck pain and whiplash.* Available from: http://www.anaes.fr/anaes/anaesparametrage.nsf/Page?ReadForm&Section=/anaes/SiteWeb.nsf/w RubriquesID/APEH-3YTFUH?OpenDocument&Defaut=y& (Accesed on 6th May 2005)

215 Bekkering, G, Hendriks HJM , Lanser K, Oostendorp RAB, Scholten-Peeters GGM, Verhagen A P and van der Windt DAWM (2003). Clinical practice guidelines for physical therapy in patients with whiplash-associated disorders. In *Clinical Practice Guidelines in the Netherlands: a prospect for continuous quality improvement in Physical Therapy.* Royal Dutch Society for Physical Therapy, Amersfoort

Further reading

The following list of textbooks were derived from the first round of the Delphi process. Specific results from Round Two can be found in Appendix H. The list is presented in order of highest to lowest Delphi scores.

Gifford, L (ed.) (1998–2002) *Topical Issues in Pain [series 1–4]*. NOI Press, Falmouth, Adelaide

Boyling, J, Palastanga, N (1994). *Grieves Modern Manual Therapy* (2nd Edition). Churchill Livingstone, Edinburgh

Main, C, Spanswick, CC (2000). *Pain Management: an Interdisciplinary Approach.* Churchill Livingstone, Edinburgh

Maitland, G, Hengerveld, E, Banks, K, English, K (2001). *Maitland's Vertebral Manipulation (6th edition).* Butterworth Heinmann, Oxford

Grieve, G P (1988). *Common Vertebral Joint Problems.* Churchill Livingstone, Edinburgh

Petty, N J, Moore, A P (2001). *Neuromusculoskeletal Examination and Assessment: A Handbook for Therapists (2nd edition)* Churchill Livingstone, Edinburgh

Grant, R (ed.) (1994). *Physical Therapy of the Cervical and Thoracic Spine (2nd edition).* Churchill Livingstone, New York

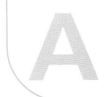

Appendix A

People involved in developing these guidelines

Table 1 The Guidelines Development Group (GDG), 2003–2004

Name	Post	Speciality
Ann Moore Ph.D., Grad. Dip. Phys., F.C.S.P., F.M.A.C.P., Dip.T.P., Cert. Ed. (Chair)	Professor of Physiotherapy, Director of Clinical Research, The University of Brighton	Musculoskeletal physiotherapy, standardised data collection & research methods
Sue Hammersley M.C.S.P.	Clinical Specialist, Calderdale & Huddersfield NHS Trust	Musculoskeletal physiotherapy outpatients
Jonathan Hill M.Sc., M.C.S.P	Research Physiotherapist, Keele University.	Musculoskeletal research
Gail Hitchcock M.Sc., MCSP	Extended Scope Physiotherapy Practitioner in Accident & Emergency, Worthing & Southlands Hospitals NHS Trust	Musculoskeletal physiotherapy
Chris Mercer M.Sc., M.M.A.C.P., M.C.S.P.	Consultant Physiotherapist, Worthing & Southlands Hospitals NHS Trust	Spinal musculoskeletal
Carole Smith M.Sc., M.M.A.C.P., M.C.S.P.	Physiotherapy Co-ordinator Musculoskeletal Services, Bradford Teaching Hospitals NHS Trust	Musculoskeletal physiotherapy
Jonathan Thompson M.C.S.P., B.H.Sc. (Hons.), M.S.O.M.	Extended Scope Practitioner, York Health Services NHS Trust	Musculoskeletal physiotherapy & orthopaedics
Martin Urmston Grad. Dip. Phys., M.C.S.P.	Physiotherapy Manager, North Manchester Health Care Trust	Musculoskeletal physiotherapy
Steve Woby Ph.D., B.Sc.(Hons.)	Research Fellow, Physiotherapy Department North Manchester General Hospital/Centre for Rehabilitation Sciences, University of Manchester	Psychosocial & cognitive behavioural interventions
Alison Hudson	Fundraising Manager, BackCare and Expert Patient	The patient's perspective
Anne Jackson Ph.D., M.Sc., M.C.S.P., B.A. (Hons.), H.T.	Guidelines Project Manager, CSP	Guideline development methods, Delphi methods, writing
Jo Jordan M.Sc., M.A., B.Sc. (Hons.)	Systematic Reviewer, CSP	Systematic review, guideline development methods, writing.
Helen Whittaker B.Sc. (Hons.)	Clinical Effectiveness Administrator, CSP	General administrative support, minutes, I.T. and data management

Table 2 The Yorkshire Steering Group (1999)

Name	Post in 1999
Jill Gregson	Physiotherapy Manager Bradford Royal Infirmary, Bradford Hospitals NHS Trust
Pam McClea	Superintendent Physiotherapist, Harrogate Health Care NHS Trust
Sue Jessop	Physiotherapy Manager, Pinderfields General Hospital, Wakefield
Jo Laycock	Independent Practitioner
Pam Janssen	Division of Physiotherapy, University of Bradford
Angela Clough	Faculty of Health and Environment, School of Health Sciences, Leeds Metropolitan University

Table 3 Yorkshire Guidelines Development Group Members (1996)

Name	Post in 1999
Group process leader	
Val Steele	Director of Rehabilitation, Bradford Hospitals NHS Trust
Group topic leaders	
Sue Hammersley	Superintendent Physiotherapist, Huddersfield NHS Trust
Jonathan Thompson	Superintendent Physiotherapist, Castle Hill Hospital, East Yorkshire Hospitals NHS Trust
Carole Smith	Superintendent Physiotherapist, Bradford Hospitals NHS Trust
Angela Clough	Faculty of Health and Environment, School of Health Sciences, Leeds Metropolitan University
Group members	
Frederique Brown	Senior I Physiotherapist, Leeds Community & Mental Health Trust
Julie Crompton	Senior I Physiotherapist, Pontefract General Hospital
Karen Hellawell	Senior I Physiotherapist, Huddersfield NHS Trust
James Milligan	Superintendent Physiotherapist, Pinderfields General Hospital, Wakefield
Julie Rogers	Superintendent Physiotherapist, Lincoln Wing, St, James's Hospital, Leeds
James Selfe	Lecturer, University of Bradford
Paul Sharples	Senior Lecturer, Leeds Metropolitan University
Vicki Stokes	Superintendent Physiotherapist, Dewsbury Health Care
Emma Summerscales	Senior II Physiotherapist, Huddersfield NHS Trust
Linda Weaver	Superintendent Physiotherapist, Scunthorpe Goole Hospitals Trust
Susan Weeks	Lecturer, University of Huddersfield
Mark Whiteley	Senior II Physiotherapist, Airedale NHS Trust
Catherine Carus	Senior I Physiotherapist, Bradford Royal Infirmary

Appendix B

Search strategies for the effectiveness of physiotherapy interventions

Original Search Strategy for the period up to 1996

The Yorkshire Group searched the following key words:

Whiplash

Cervical spine

Physio/physical therapy

Management/evaluation/intervention/treatment

Education/advice/collars/prophylaxis

Exercise/mobilisation/manipulation

Compensation

Prognosis

Chronic Pain/whiplash

Pain/whiplash

Acute pain/whiplash

The original search was carried out through the Chartered Society of Physiotherapy (CSP) database and searched the following indices:

Physiotherapy Index (1986–1996)

Rehabilitation Index (1987–1996)

Complementary Medicine Index (1985–1996)

Occupational Therapy Index (1986–1996)

MEDLINE (Index Medicus, 1986–1996)

CINAHL (Cumulative Index to Nursing and Allied Health 1983–1996)

ASSIA (Applied Social Sciences Index and Abstracts 1987–1996)

CSP Physiotherapy Research Projects Database

CSP Physiotherapy Documents Database

WCPT proceedings (1995 only)

The Cochrane Database of Systematic Reviews

The Database of Abstracts of Reviews of Effectiveness

EMBASE

AMED

BIDS (Includes psychology journals)

The time period over which databases were searched was determined by the parameters of the CSP's database.

Search strategy for period 1995 to January 2001

The keywords 'whiplash' or 'whiplash injuries' were searched (or mapped to search terms and expanded where available) on the following databases: Medline, CINAHL, AMED, Science Citation Index (SCI), Social Science Citation Index (SSCI), BIDS, and EDINA Ei Compendex. In addition, 'cervical spine' was combined with other keywords 'manual therapy', 'mobilisation', 'mobilization', 'traction', 'exercise', 'physiotherapy', 'physical therapy', 'electrotherapy', 'laser', 'ultrasound', 'electrical stimulation', 'short wave', 'collars', 'joint instability' on Medline, CINAHL and AMED.

Proceedings from IFOMT, MPAA and WCPT conferences were also hand searched from 1996 to 2001.

Update searches after January 2001

A keyword search for 'whiplash' on Medline, CINAHL, AMED, SCI, SSCI, The Cochrane Library, PEDro, Applied Social Science Index and Abstracts, & Expanded Academic Index was carried out for the update searches. Databases were searched from 1995 if they had not been included in previous searches.

Final update search strategies February/March 2004

MEDLINE

Limits English language, human, 2001 –

Keywords:

whiplash OR whiplash injuries

OR

cervical vertebrae subheadings injuries OR physiopathology AND (neck injuries subheadings diagnosis, etiology, physiopathology, rehabilitation, therapy OR manipulation spinal OR physical therapy techniques OR exercise therapy OR movement OR early ambulation OR traction OR electric stimulation OR electric stimulation therapy OR laser therapy low level OR deceleration OR acceleration OR ultrasonics OR short wave therapy OR orthotic devices OR joint instability)

EMBASE – Physical Medicine and Rehabilitation

Limits English Language, 1995 –

Keywords:

whiplash OR whiplash injuries

OR

(cervical spine injury OR neck pain) AND (traction therapy OR physiotherapy OR manipulative medicine OR chiropractic spinal manipulation OR spinal manipulation OR electrostimulation OR orthoses OR spine stabilization OR ultrasound therapy OR low level laser therapy OR joint instability)

AMED

Limits English Language, 2001 –

Keywords:

whiplash OR whiplash injuries

OR

(neck injuries OR cervical vertebrae) AND (manipulation OR chiropractic OR manipulation, osteopathic OR musculoskeletal manipulations OR spinal manipulation OR physiotherapy OR physiotherapy methods OR movement OR early ambulation OR traction OR electric stimulation OR electroacupuncture OR transcutaneous electric nerve stimulation OR laser therapy low level OR acceleration OR ultrasonics OR orthotic devices OR short wave diathermy OR joint instability)

CINAHL

Limits English Language, 2001 –

Keywords:

whiplash OR whiplash injuries

OR

(cervical vertebrae subheadings injuries or physiopathology OR neck injuries subheadings etiology or physiopathology or rehabilitation or therapy) AND (physical therapy OR manual therapy OR therapeutic exercise OR movement OR early ambulation OR traction OR electric stimulation OR electric stimulation functional OR electric stimulation neuromuscular OR lasers OR ultrasonics OR diathermy OR orthoses OR orthoses design OR joint instability)

Also searched the following databases for keyword 'whiplash'

PEDro Database

The Cochrane Library, 2004 issue 1 (Cochrane Database of Systematic Reviews and DARE)

Hand search of IFOMT 7th conference proceedings (2000) incorporating the 11th MPAA conference and 12th MPA conference available from
http://www.physiotherapy.asn.au/conferences/proceedings/Table%20of%20Contents.pdf

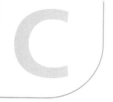

Appendix C

Evidence tables of studies included in the evidence review

Appendix C includes:

Table 1   Evidence table of the 12 RCTs relating to WAD included in the evidence review and one RCT relating to chronic neck pain

Table 2   Evidence table of systematic reviews on non-specific neck pain

Table 3   Evidence table of systematic reviews on WAD, which were used to identify relevant individual studies

Table 1 Evidence table of the 12 RCTs relating to WAD included in the evidence review and one RCT relating to chronic neck pain

Reference	Methodological quality	Interventions
Bonk et al, 2000[32]	**Eligibility?** Yes **Random?** Yes **Concealed?** No **Baseline?** Yes **Blind subjects?** No **Blind therapists?** No **Blind assessment?** No **85% follow up?** Yes **ITT?** No **Groups compared?** Yes **Points & variation?** Yes **Score: 5/10**	**Group A (n=47): Active therapy** – 3 sessions first week & 2 in each of next 2 weeks. In each session ice applied for 10 minutes, mobilisation by therapist through full tolerable range of motion with patient, followed by active mobilisation by patient as described in study by Mealy and then strengthening & isometric exercises. First week in supine position, second week patient seated. In third week patient given interscapular muscle strengthening exercises & advice on maintaining normal posture. Told not to use a collar. **Group B (n=50): Collar** – Asked to wear a collar for 3 weeks during day. Given no physiotherapy, activity, exercises or mobilisation. Both groups could use analgesics or anti-inflammatories as they wished. **Group C (n=50): Healthy subjects** – comparison group

Participants	Outcomes	Results (incl. withdrawals)	Conclusions & comments
Country: Germany **Setting of study:** Emergency department **Inclusion:** Accident victims of rear-end collisions, between 16 & 60 years old & within 3 days of accident **Exclusion:** prior neurological disease, prior neck injury, x-rays showing old fractures or skeletal malformations, spondyloarthropathy, symptom onset more than 3 days after accident & grade 3 or 4 whiplash-associated disorder.	**Follow up:** 12 weeks **Outcomes:** Neck pain, neck stiffness, headache, shoulder pain, arm pain & neck ROM. Neck mobility measured in flexion/extension by difference between smallest & greatest distance of chin to sternal notch. Lateral flexion & rotation measured with goniometer. Left & right side angles added to provide total lateral flexion.	**6 (4%) withdrawals, all from group A** **Neck pain:** Onset: 98% group A, 96% Group B & 8% Group C. 6 weeks: 11% Group A, 62% Group B. 12 weeks: 2% Group A, 16% Group B. **Flexion/extension [mean(SD)].** 19.9cm(1.8) Healthy group. 6 weeks: 19.2 (2.0)cm Group A, 17.7 (4.6)cm Group B. 12 weeks: 19.4 (1.8) Group A, 18.3 (1.6)cm Group B. **Lateral flexion [mean(SD)].** 88.1(4.4)° Healthy group. 6 weeks: 89.8(6.6)° Group A, 82.5(6.5)° Group B. 12 weeks: 88.3(4.2)° Group A, 85.7(4.9)° Group B. **Rotation [mean(SD)]:** 178.2(5.3)° Healthy group. 6 weeks: 176.9(8.0)° Group A, 165.1(16.7)° Group B. 12 weeks: 178.5(4.6)° Group A, 175.4(8.1)° Group B.	Study confirms that active therapy compared to use of collar and rest results in significant difference in rate of recovery. **Comments** Not sure if differences sig. or if intention-to-treat analysis used. Only measured healthy group once and everything compared to their initial results.

Reference	Methodological quality	Interventions
Borchgrevnik et al, 1998 [33]	**Eligibility?** Yes **Random?** Yes **Concealed?** No **Baseline?** Yes **Blind subjects?** No **Blind therapists?** No **Blind assessment?** Yes **85% follow up?** Yes **ITT?** No **Groups compared?** Yes **Points & variation?** Yes **Score: 6/10**	**Group A (n=82): Act as usual** – instructed to act as usual with no sick leave or collar **Group B (n=96): Immobilisation** – 14 days sick leave and immobilised with a soft neck collar for 14 days (alternating 2 hours on & 2 hours off & continuously at night)
Fitz-Ritson, 1995 [34]	**Eligibility?** No **Random?** Yes **Concealed?** No **Baseline?** No **Blind subjects?** No **Blind therapists?** No **Blind assessment?** No **85% follow up?** Yes **ITT?** No **Groups compared?** No **Points & variation?** Yes **Score: 3/10**	Both groups continued with chiropractic treatments. Each group did a series of exercises for 8 weeks, 5 days per week. **Group A (n=15):** 4 levels (10 exercises in each) with 2 weeks on each level. Levels: a) range of motion, b) stretching, c) isometric-toning & d) isokinetic-strengthening **Group B (n=15):** phasic neck exercises – 2 levels (8 exercises in each) with 4 weeks on each level. For example, Level 1, exercise 1: lying, rotate the eyes and head to same side; exercise 2: lying?, rotate eyes & head to the same side. Level 2, exercise 7: moving eye-head-neck-arm in coordinated pattern; exercise 8: rotate eye-head-neck-trunk, looking as far behind as possible.

Participants	Outcomes	Results (incl. withdrawals)	Conclusions & comments
Country: Norway **Setting of study:** Emergency clinic **Inclusion criteria:** Patients with neck sprain injury caused by private car accident with reported material damage from rear-end, side- or head-on collisions, aged between 18 and 70 years. **Exclusion criteria:** Patients in bus or large-vehicle accidents; radiographically disclosed vertebral fractures; clinical signs of nerve root compression; simultaneous concussion or other head trauma; & those who lived too far from centre.	**Follow up:** 14 days, 6 weeks & 6 months – questionnaires & physical examinations. **Outcomes:** Post-intervention: Patients' subjective symptoms related to neck injury; Neurologic investigation; Neck movement – using instrument like the Cybex Model DEI-320; Shoulder movement. At 2 & 6 weeks and 6 months after accident: neck pain (VAS), neck stiffness & headache (VAS) Also measured shoulder pain, back pain, chest pain, difficulties with memory, difficulties with concentration, buzzing ears, dizziness, nausea, diminished vision, insomnia, analgesia, depression & anxiety.	23 (14 group A & 9 group B) dropped out & did not attend at 6 months. Also incomplete questionnaires: 16 at intake, 10 at 6 weeks & 15 at 6 months. Neck pain (VAS) **Baseline:** 33.0 ± 2.5 group A & 38.1 ± 2.6 group B. **6 weeks:** 32.9 ± 3.9 group A & 29.7 ± 2.7 group B. **6 months:** 26.6 ± 2.6 group A & 31.1 ±3.2 group B. Headache (VAS) **Baseline:** 24.2 ± 2.7 group A & 33.3 ± 3.0 group B. **6 weeks:** 28.2 ± 3.6 group A & 27.8 ± 3.0 group B. **6 months:** 21.4 ± 3.4 group A & 33.2 ± 3.2 group B. 8 (10%) group A & 7 (7%) group B on sick leave at 6 months. **Global improvement:** More symptoms: 17 (21%) group A & 21 (22%) group B. As before: 11 (13%) group A & 14 (15%) group B. Less symptoms: 54(66%) & 60 (63%) group B. 20% in both groups reported feeling worse at 6 months than at 14 days after accident. No difference between groups in either neck or shoulder movements at either 14 days or 6 months	Patients who were instructed to continue engaging in their normal activities (act as usual) after neck sprain injury had a better outcome than patients who took sick leave from work and who were immobilised with soft neck collars during the first 14 days after the accident. **Comments** Differences at baseline in neck pain VAS mean little difference in improvement between 2 groups. No intention-to-treat, several incomplete questionnaires at each follow up, but don't know from which group.
Country: Canada **Setting of study:** clinic **Inclusion criteria:** Patients with pain 12 weeks after vehicle accident; increased pain/soreness/stiffness of cervical musculature with sport or activity requiring rapid neck movements. **Exclusion criteria:** None given.	**Follow up:** 8 weeks, administered by receptionist. **Outcomes:** Neck Pain Disability Index.	None lost to follow up or withdrawn from study. Average pre-therapy NPDI: 59.5 group A vs. 60 group B. Average post-therapy NPDI: 55.1 group A vs. 31 group B.	It has been shown that a phasic component to neck movement and its restoration seems to be important in the rehabilitation of the injured cervical spine. **Comments** Groups not compared with each other. Baseline differences in groups in age, number of patients having >1 accident, gender.

Reference	Methodological quality	Interventions
Foley-Nolan et al, 1992 [35]	**Eligibility?** Yes **Random?** Yes **Concealed?** Yes **Baseline?** No **Blind subjects?** Yes **Blind therapists?** Yes **Blind assessment?** Yes **85% follow up?** Yes **ITT?** Yes **Groups compared?** Yes **Points & variation?** Yes **Score: 9/10**	**Group A (n=20):** Active PEMT unit consisting of soft collar containing flexible miniaturised short wave diathermy generator (100gms weight). Generator produced pulsed magnetic field in treatment area with mean power 1.5 mWatts/cm^2 at patient's surface. Nominal frequency of unit was 27MHz, with pulsed burst width 60 microseconds and repetition frequency of 450 per second. Each unit had on/off switch & light to confirm system operational. Powered by two 9 volt batteries replaced at 4 weeks. **Group B (n=20):** Dummy unit with generator of same weight incorporated but not producing PEMT waves. Also had on/off switch & indicator light and was battery operated. Each unit had identity number and only agent of manufacturer (H & K Electronics) knew which were active. Collars to be worn 8 hours per day for the 12 weeks of study. NSAIDs prescribed and amount taken recorded. Patients advised to mobilise neck hourly with each of 6 cervical movements 5 times each within pain-free range. If unhappy with progress at 4 weeks referred to physio for 2 sessions per week for 6 weeks tailored to individual needs (typically included hot pack, pulsed short wave diathermy, ultrasound & active repetitive movements).
Gennis et al, 1996 [36]	**Eligibility?** Yes **Random?** No **Concealed?** No **Baseline?** Yes **Blind subjects?** No **Blind therapists?** No **Blind assessment?** No **85% follow up?** No **ITT?** No **Groups compared?** Yes **Points & variation?** Yes **Score: 3/10**	**Group A (n=104):** Universal Cervical Collar (Star Manufacturers, LA, USA) – foam rubber collar with Velcro fastener allowing 1-size to fit all adults. Instructed to wear as much as could in first 2 weeks after injury. **Group B (n=92):** Control Group. Both groups advised to rest and given analgesics (usually NSAIDs) at discretion of treating physician.

Participants	Outcomes	Results (incl. withdrawals)	Conclusions & comments
Country: Ireland **Setting of study:** A & E Dept **Inclusion criteria:** Patients over 18 years old with acute whiplash injuries from rear-end collisions. **Exclusion criteria:** Presenting at A & E >72 hours after injury; active inflammatory, infective, neoplastic, or metastatic bone disease involving cervical spine; cervical fracture; head injury with loss of consciousness; impaired reflexes indicative of cervical root lesion.	**Follow up:** 2, 4 & 12 weeks **Outcomes:** Pain: 10cm VAS. Range of neck movement: graded as full, 2/3 normal, 1/3 normal or absent (max. 6 pts total ROM). Subjective assessment of progress: patients perceived progress, 9-pt scale: worst possible, much worse, moderately worse, mildly worse, no change, mildly better, moderately better, much better and completely well.	None lost to follow up Neck pain VAS (mean?): baseline, 6.75 group A vs. 6.25 group B (NS); 4 weeks, 2.5 group A vs. 5.00 group B (p<0.05); 12 weeks, 1.5 group A vs. 2.25 group B (NS). Neck movement (??): baseline, 2.83 group A vs. 3.66 group B (p<0.05); 4 weeks, 4.0 group A vs. 3.33 group B (NS); 12 weeks, 4.5 group A vs. 4.00 group B (p<0.05). Patient perceived improvement as 'moderately' or 'much' better: 4 weeks, 17(85%) group A vs. 7 (35%) group B (p=0.001); 12 weeks, 85% group A vs. 60% group B.	The significant patient improvement as judged by both patient in terms of pain and subjective assessment and clinician in terms of ROM, strongly suggests that PEMT has a beneficial effect in the early management of acute whiplash injury. **Comments**
Country: USA **Setting of study:** Adult emergency dept of urban, level I trauma centre. **Inclusion criteria:** Patients presenting with neck pain less than 24 hours after a motor vehicle crash. **Exclusion criteria:** Patients with fractures or dislocations of cervical spine, focal neurological findings (central or peripheral) or other injuries that might distract attention from neck pain, those requiring hospitalisation or with impaired cognitive function precluding informed consent.	**Follow up:** 6 weeks **Outcomes:** Initial data – contact details, age, gender, seat position in car, seat belt use, medications prescribed, initial pain on 100mm VAS Follow up data – date of contact, degree of pain (none, better, same, worse), further care received, days & hours per day of collar use & whether patient felt better when wearing the collar.	54 of original 250 people not attending at 6 weeks. **At 6 weeks** No pain: 43/104 in group A & 31/92 in group B. Pain 'better': 46/104 in group A & 42/92 in group B. Pain 'same': 10/104 in group A & 12/92 in group B. Pain 'worse': 5/104 in group A & 7/92 in group B. Of 86 (83%) of soft collar wearers expressing a preference, 68 (79%) said the collar provided some degree of pain relief.	Most patients with whiplash injury can expect to have pain for >6 weeks. Soft cervical collars do not affect the severity or duration of pain >=6 weeks post-injury. **Comments**

Reference	Methodological quality	Interventions
Irnich et al, 2001 [154]	**Eligibility?** Yes **Random?** Yes **Concealed?** No **Baseline?** Yes **Blind subjects?** No **Blind therapists?** No **Blind assessment?** Yes **85% follow up?** Yes **ITT?** No **Groups compared?** Yes **Points & variation?** Yes **Score:** 7/10	**Group A (n=56): Acupuncture** – according to traditional Chinese medicine rules, including diagnostic palpation for sensitive spots. **Group B (n=60): Massage** – conventional Western massage, including effleurage, petrissage, friction, tapotement & vibration. Did not include spinal manipulation or non-conventional techniques. **Group C (n=61): Placebo** – sham laser acupuncture with laser pen (Seirin International, Fort Lauderdale, USA) emitting only red light, accompanied by visual & acoustic signals. Diagnostic palpation same as for acupuncture group.
McKinney et al, 1989 [38,39]	**Eligibility?** Yes **Random?** Yes **Concealed?** No **Baseline?** Yes **Blind subjects?** No **Blind therapists?** No **Blind assessment?** Yes **85% follow up?** No **ITT?** No **Groups compared?** Yes **Points & variation?** Yes **Score:** 5/10	All fitted with soft foam collar and given analgesic (co-dydramol 1,000 mg 6-hourly). **Group A (n=33): Rest** – general advice to mobilise after initial rest period of 10–14 days. **Group B (n=71): Physiotherapy** – assessed by physiotherapist and tailored programme devised from resources available at the hospital. Typically, combination of hot & cold applications, pulsed short wave diathermy, hydrotherapy, traction, & active & passive repetitive movements. Each patient had 10 hours of physiotherapy over 6 weeks. **Group C (n=66): Advice** – assessed by physiotherapist & given verbal and reinforcing written instruction on correct posture, use of analgesia and collar, and on use of heat sources and muscle relaxation. Encourage to perform mobilising exercises that were demonstrated. Emphasis on maintaining good range of neck movements and on correcting posture even if initially causes more discomfort. Advised to restrict use of collar to short periods when neck vulnerable to sudden jolting. Session lasted typically 30 minutes.

Participants	Outcomes	Results (incl. withdrawals)	Conclusions & comments
Country: Germany **Setting of study:** out-patient departments. **Inclusion criteria:** Patients with painful restriction of cervical spine mobility for more than 1 month & no treatment in 2 weeks before entering study. **Exclusion criteria:** previous surgery, dislocation, fracture, neurological deficits, systemic disorders or contraindications to treatment.	**Follow up:** Immediately & 3 days after first treatment and immediately & a week after last treatment. Followed up at 3 months. **Primary outcome:** Change in maximum pain related to motion in most affected direction (100 point VAS). **Secondary outcomes:** Active ROM (3D ultrasound real time motion analyser (Zebris Medizinintechnik, Germany). Intensity of direction related pain assessed by patient (VAS). Pressure pain threshold bilaterally at 3 sites & individual maximum point using digital pressure algometer. Changes in spontaneous pain, motion related pain & global complaints (7 pt scale). SF-36 health survey.	12 withdrawn (5 group A, 3 group B & 4 group C). Mean improvement in VAS pain at 1 week: 24.22 (16.5-31.9) Group A, 7.89 (0.6-15.2) Group B, 17.28 (10.0-24.6) Group C. Sig difference group A vs. group B. Not sig. group A vs. group C. Differences between groups more distinct in subgroup who had myofascial pain & those who had pain > 5 years. Acupuncture group had best results in secondary outcomes immediately and 1 week after therapy, but no longer significant after 3 months. Quality of life measures improved in all groups, but no significant difference between groups. Side effects: 17 (33%) reported mild reactions during acupuncture, slight pain or vegetative reactions. Mild reactions also in 4 (7%) of massage group and 12 (21%) in sham laser group. No serious adverse reactions reported.	Trial showed that acupuncture is a safe and effective form of treatment for people with chronic neck pain. Effects on pain and mobility were better than those achieved with conventional massage.
Country: Northern Ireland **Setting of study:** A & E dept. **Inclusion criteria:** Patients with whiplash injury within 48 hours of road accident. **Exclusion criteria:** Radiological or clinical evidence of fracture or dislocation or pre-existing degenerative diseases.	**Follow up:** 1,2 & 3 months & 2 years. **Outcomes:** Pain 10cm VAS. ROM.	Randomisation to the group allocated 'rest' stopped early in trial for ethical reasons. Neck pain (median VAS): baseline, 5.6 group A, 5.32 group B & 5.3 group C; 1 month, 4.97 group A, 3.28 group B & 3.37 group C; 2 months, 3.0 group A, 1.94 group B & 1.82 group C. Lateral flexion ROM [mean (SD)]: baseline, 44.4 (14.7) group A, 45.6 (18.5) group B & 47.3 (20.7) group C; 1 month, 41.8 (18.9) group A, 53.3 (20.3) group B & 54.1 (19.7) group C; 2 months, 55.1 (14.8) group A, 64.0 (12.9) group B & 64.1 (12.7) group C. Those available at 2 years: 12 (46%) group A, 24 (44%) group B & 11 (23%) group C had persistent symptoms.	At 2 months there appeared to be no difference in the effectiveness between out-patient physiotherapy and home mobilisation. Advice to mobilise in the early phase after neck injury reduces the number of patients with symptoms at two years and is superior to manipulative physiotherapy. Prolonged wearing of a collar is associated with persistence of symptoms. **Comments**

Reference	Methodological quality	Interventions
Mealy et al, 1986[40]	**Eligibility?** No **Random?** Yes **Concealed?** Yes **Baseline?** Yes **Blind subjects?** No **Blind therapists?** No **Blind assessment?** Yes **85% follow up?** Yes **ITT?** No **Groups compared?** Yes **Points & variation?** Yes **Score: 6/10**	**Group A (n=31):** Active treatment – applications of ice in first 24 hours then neck mobilisation using Maitland technique and daily exercises of cervical spine. Maitland technique – repetitive & passive movements within patient's tolerance, movements with small amplitude for pain & spasm & with larger amplitude for stiffness. Local heat applied after each treatment. Daily exercises performed every hour at home, within limits of pain. **Group B (n=30):** Standard treatment – soft cervical collar & advised to rest for 2 weeks before starting gradual mobilisation. All patients received analgesics as required.
Pennie & Agambar, 1990[41]	**Eligibility?** Yes **Random?** No **Concealed?** No **Baseline?** No **Blind subjects?** No **Blind therapists?** No **Blind assessment?** No **85% follow up?** Yes **ITT?** No **Groups compared?** Yes **Points & variation?** Yes **Score: 3/10**	**Group A (n=74):** Collar – standard treatment of 2 weeks rest in either soft collar or moulded thermoplastic polyethylene foam. Patients reviewed & taught programme of active exercises. At 6–8 weeks those who did not improve or deteriorated were referred for physio. **Group B (n=61):** Traction – active treatment by traction and exercises. Patients attended twice per week and had intermittent halter traction for 10 minutes: 12 lb (5.4kg) applied for 30 seconds with 30 second rest periods. Traction applied in extension, neutral position or flexion for upper, mid or lower neck pain respectively. Patients had advice on neck care & sleeping posture & between attendances asked to perform simple neck & shoulder exercises.

Participants	Outcomes	Results (incl. withdrawals)	Conclusions & comments
Country: Ireland **Setting of study:** A & E Dept. **Inclusion criteria:** Patients with acute whiplash injuries within 24 hours of accident. **Exclusion criteria:** Cervical fractures.	**Follow up:** 4, 8 weeks after accident. **Outcomes:** Pain VAS. Cervical movement.	10 withdrawn from study, 5 in each in group. Neck pain [mean VAS (SEM)]: baseline, 5.71 (0.44) group A & 6.44 (0.41) group B; 4 weeks, 2.85 (0.57) group A vs. 5.08(0.48) group B (p<0.05); 8 weeks, 1.69(0.43) group A vs. 3.94(0.58) group B (p<0.0125). ROM [mean (SEM)]: baseline, 19.92 (1.74) group A vs. 25.00 (2.17) group B; 4 weeks, 29.03 (2.12) group A vs. 27.56 (2.09) group B; 8 weeks, 34.11 (1.5) group A vs. 29.57 (1.61) group B (p<0.05).	Results confirmed expectations that initial immobility after whiplash injuries gives rise to prolonged symptoms, whereas a more rapid improvement can be achieved by early active management without any consequent increase in discomfort. **Comments** Only 8 week follow up.
Country: England **Setting of study:** Research clinic. **Inclusion criteria:** Patients with soft tissue injury of the neck sustained in road traffic accidents. **Exclusion criteria:** None given.	**Follow up:** continued until patient felt recovered or up to 5 months later. Non-attendees visited at home 5 months after injury. **Outcomes:** Total neck mobility – measured in degrees on goniometer as sum of flexion, extension, left & right lateral flexion and left & right rotation. Pain – four sites (neck, arm, back, & head) using 100-pt VAS	3 from group A excluded from both assessments, 23 from 6-8 week & 20 from 5 month reviews. Average % reduction neck pain VAS (no. of patients): 6-8 weeks, 64 (61) group A & 68 (48) group B; 5 months, 88 (70) group A & 90 (58) group B. Total movement [mean (range)]: baseline, 288 (85-455) group A & 276 (85-425) group B; 6-8 weeks, 361 (190-460) group A & 366 (140-470) group B; 5 months, 377 (190-460) group A & 366 (140-470) group B. Average days off work [mean (median)]: 26 (17) group A & 31 (11) group B out of 57 people in group A & 48 in group B.	We cannot recommend the use of the active treatment we have described, and feel that any alternative should be rigorously evaluated because of the expense and resources involved. **Comments** Not true randomisation.

Reference	Methodological quality	Interventions
Provinciali et al, 1996 [42]	**Eligibility?** Yes **Random?** Yes **Concealed?** No **Baseline?** Yes **Blind subjects?** No **Blind therapists?** No **Blind assessment?** Yes **85% follow up?** Yes **ITT?** No **Groups compared?** Yes **Points & variation?** Yes **Score: 6/10**	**Group A (n=30):** Multimodal treatment: – Relaxation training based on diaphragmatic breathing in supine position; - Active reduction of cervical & lumbar lordosis, based on suggestions provided by Neck School (Sweeney, 1992). - Psychological support to reduce anxiety & limit emotional influence (Radanov, 1991). - Eye fixation exercises in order to prevent dizziness, according to technique (Shutty, 1991). - Manual treatment (massage, mobilisation) of cervical spine. **Group B (n=30):** Physical agents: TENS (especially applied to Arnold's nerve) & PEMT (Foley-Nolan, 1990), and Ultrasound (1.5 Watt/cm^2) and calcic iontophoresis with calcium chloride (Foreman, 1995). Each patient had 10, 1-hour treatment sessions over two-week peroid.
Rosenfeld et al, 2000 [43]	**Eligibility?** Yes **Random?** Yes **Concealed?** No **Baseline?** Yes **Blind subjects?** No **Blind therapists?** No **Blind assessment?** No **85% follow up?** Yes **ITT?** No **Groups compared?** Yes **Points & variation?** No **Score: 4/10**	**Group A (n=21): Active 96hrs** – active exercise & posture protocol consistent with McKenzie's principles. Gentle, active, small-range & amplitude rotational movements of neck, repeated 10 times in both directions every waking hour. Movements made to maximum comfortable range. Patients taught to recognise warning signs & adjust amplitude and/or number of movements. Treated within 96 hours of trauma, reassessed after 20 days using dynamic mechanical evaluation consistent with McKenzie protocol. Individual program added if symptoms persisted (cervical retraction, extension, flexion, rotation, lateral flexion or combination of these depending which were beneficial during assessment). **Group B (n=23): Standard 96 hrs** – Leaflet with info on injury mechanisms, advice on suitable activities & postural correction given within 96 hours of trauma. Advised to rest neck during first weeks after injury and that wearing soft collar could provide comfort & prevent excessive movement. Also advised to begin performing active movements 2 or 3 times a day a few weeks after injury. **Group C (n=22): Active 14 days** – as Group A with delay 14 days. **Group D (n=22): Standard 14 days** – as Group B with delay 14 days.

Participants	Outcomes	Results (incl. withdrawals)	Conclusions & comments
Country: Italy Setting of study: Not given Inclusion criteria: Patients with "neck sprain" following car accident; within 60 days of injury; regular performance of job or profession before accident. Exclusion criteria: Infective, neoplastic, metabolic or inflammatory bone disease; x-ray evidence of traumatic or severe degenerative lesions of cervical spine; symptom exaggeration with intention of enhancing financial rewards.	Follow up: Assessment before, immediately after treatment, one & 6 months after baseline assessment. Outcomes: Cervical ROM – maximal flexion, declination & rotation in ordinal scale (0 to 6). Pain – 10 pt VAS. Self-rating scale – subjective judgement of changes from baseline (+3:total recovery; +2:marked improvement; +1:slight improvement; 0: no change; -1:slight impairment; -2: marked impairment; -3:complete disability). Return to work – time from injury to return to work.	Median ROM: baseline, 3.8 group A vs. 3.9 group B; 6 months, 5.5 group A vs. 4.6 group B. Pain (median VAS): 6.8 group A vs. 7.4 group B; 6 months, 1.9 group A vs. 4.8 group B. Self-rating scale (median): post-therapy, 1 group A vs. 0 group B; 6 months, 2 group A vs. −1 group B. 29/30 in group A & 24/30 in group B returned to work by 6 months. Mean (SD) delay in returning to work, 38.4 (10.5) group A & 54.3 (18.4) in group B.	Results confirm hypothesis of multifactorial involvement as a possible mechanism for the late whiplash syndrome. Comments
Country: Sweden Setting of study: 29 primary care units, 3 emergency wards & several private clinics referred patients to the study. Inclusion: acute whiplash injury caused by motor vehicle accident within 96 hours of trauma. Exclusion: cervical fractures, cervical dislocation, head injury, previous symptomatic chronic neck problems, alcohol abuse, dementia, serious mental diseases or diseases likely to cause death before the end of the study.	Follow up: 6 months Outcomes: Range of motion measured by medical lab technologist or registered nurse. Cervical measurement system used to measure lateral flexion, extension-flexion & rotation using an inclinometer & compass for rotation. Pain measured on VAS.	9 (9%) withdrawals, don't know which groups. Change in mean pain VAS: -30 Group A, +0.74 Group B, -15 Group C & -7.1 Group D (sig. difference between groups). No pain (VAS=0): 8 (38%) Group A, 4 (17%) Group B, 5 (23%) Group C & 1 (5%) Group D. Low pain (VAS<=10): 11 (52%) Group A, 7 (30%) Group B, 8 (36%) Group C & 2 (9%) Group D. Change in mean total ROM: +51.9 Group A, +26.2 Group B, +23.3 Group C & +44.6 Group D (no sig. difference between groups). Combined time & treatment effect on pain.	Early treatment with frequently repeated active submaximal movements combined with mechanical diagnosis & therapy is more effective in reducing pain than treatment with initial rest, recommendation of soft collar and a gradual introduction of home exercises. Comments Not sure if differences sig. or if intention-to-treat analysis used. Study complicated by 4-group design.

Reference	Methodological quality	Interventions
Soderlund, 2000[44]	**Eligibility?** Yes **Random?** Yes **Concealed?** No **Baseline?** Yes **Blind subjects?** No **Blind therapists?** No **Blind assessment?** No **85% follow up?** No **ITT?** No **Groups compared?** Yes **Points & variation?** Yes **Score: 4/10**	**Group A (n=26): Regular treatment** – 3 exercises at least 3 times per day, cautiously until pain limit reached to restore normal neck movements: 1) looking over each shoulder in turn, 3–5 times; 2) moving arms up and down anteriorly, 2–3 times; 3) taking deep breath & lifting shoulders upwards exhaling & relaxing shoulders. Advised to alternate rest & activities, keep neck warm, walk fair distance every day & keep upright posture when sitting, standing or walking, instructed not to lift or carry heavy objects & not to remain seated with head bent forward in first weeks after injury. Only to use a collar if traveling extensively or reading/studying for several hours per day. **Group B (n=27): Additional treatment** – Same as regular group with added exercise to improve kinaesthetic sensibility & coordination of neck muscles. Exercise taught with patient lying on floor, asked to imagine a 'quadrangle' under head and to gently press each angle of the 'quadrangle', one at a time against floor. Cycle repeated 3 times. Patients then asked to press 2 diagonal angles towards surface at same time, 3 times. Exercise done at least 3 times a day.

Methodological Quality Assessment: PEDro Scale[45]

Criteria	Key
1. Eligibility criteria specified?	Eligibility?
2. Random allocation of participants to groups?	Random?
3. Allocation concealed?	Concealed?
4. Groups similar at baseline for most important prognostic factors?	Baseline?
5. Blinding of participants?	Blind subjects?
6. Blinding of those administering therapy?	Blind therapists?
7. Blinding of outcome assessors?	Blind assessment?
8. Follow up of more than 85% of participants initially allocated to groups?	85% follow up?
9. Intention-to-treat analysis used?	ITT?
10. Between group statistical comparisons reported?	Groups compared?
11. Point and variability measures given?	Points & variation?

Score out of 10, items 2 to 11 (item 1 not included, as this indicates external, and other items measure internal, validity)

Participants	Outcomes	Results (incl. withdrawals)	Conclusions & comments
Country: Sweden **Setting of study:** Emergency department. **Inclusion:** Patients with acute whiplash & report of acceleration-deceleration movement of head without direct head trauma. Also aged between 18 & 60 years & good ability to understand written Swedish. **Exclusion:** Previous history of neck injury due to accident.	**Follow up:** 6 months. **Outcomes:** Pain – Pain Disability Index (PDI) & VAS. Self-efficacy Scale. Coping Strategies Questionnaire. Diaries of exercise to determine compliance. Cervicothoracic posture – universal goniometer. Cervical range of motion – Lic Rehab Care. Svetsary goniometer Cervicocephalic kinaesthetic sensibility.	13 (20%) withdrawals, 6 group A & 7 group B. Compliance poor – 41% completed exercises >5 days per week. **Pain mean (SD) VAS.** 3 months: 2.2 (2.0) Group A, 2.6 (2.4) Group B. 6 months: 2.0 (1.7) Group A, 1.8 (1.9) Group B. **Left rotation mean (SD) ROM.** 3 months: 59.9 (12.9) Group A, 67.4 (11.1) Group B. 6 months: 60.3 (12.9) Group A, 69.0 (11.6) Group B. **Right rotation mean (SD) ROM.** 3 months: 59.7 (14.8) Group A, 60.9 (12.2) Group B. 6 months: 60.6 (12.4) Group A, 63.9 (13.0) Group B.	Small number of common exercises, done regularly, seem to be sufficient treatment for some patients with acute WAD. More supervision during first weeks might increase compliance. Patients' perceived disability & confidence in completing daily activities important factors in long-term symptomatology. **Comments** Not sure if differences sig. or if intention-to-treat analysis used. Poor compliance may also have effect on results.

Table 2. Evidence table of systematic reviews on non-specific neck pain

Reference	Patients	Interventions	Study designs
Albright et al, 2001[150]	**Include:** Patients with non-specific neck pain with or without pain radiating to extremities. **Exclude:** studies with mixed acute & chronic neck pain.	**Include:** massage, thermal therapy (hot or cold packs), electrical stimulation, electromyographic (EMG) biofeedback, TENS, therapeutic ultrasound, therapeutic exercises, & combinations. Control groups with active interventions & concurrent interventions if given same way to both groups. **Exclude:** concurrent interventions not given same way to experimental & control groups.	**Include:** RCTs, CCTs, case control or cohort studies of >10 subjects, written in English, French or Spanish languages. **Exclude:** Abstracts only.

Outcomes	Search strategy	Results	Conclusions

Include: Functional status, pain, ability to work, patient global improvement, patient satisfaction, quality of life.

Medline, Embase, Current contents, CINAHL, CCTR – all searched to 1st July 2000.
Register of Cochrane Rehabilitation & Related Therapies Field & Cochrane Musculoskeletal Group and PEDro. Reference lists screened, content experts contacted.

Acute

Manual Traction: Pennie 1990 & British Assoc. of Physical Medicine 1966 excluded.

TENS (Level I - RCT): Nordemar 1981 – RCT; N=20; 1) TENS (15 mins, 3 per wk at 0.2 milliseconds, 80Hz) vs. 2) Collar (<3 days); no neurological signs; No difference in patient-assessed pain after 1 wk or 3 months.

Interventions where no evidence found: EMG biofeedback, thermotherapy, massage, electrical stimulation, therapeutic exercises, or combined interventions. Mealy 1986, Borchgrevink 1998 & McKinney 1989 excluded.

Chronic

Therapeutic exercises (Level I - RCT): Vasseljen 1995, Friedrich 1996, Fitz-Ritson 1995 & Taimela 2000 excluded.

Goldie 1970 – CCT; N=47; sig. clinically important patient global improvement in isometric exercise group over no treatment group, relative risk difference 41%.

Group fitness classes: 2 RCTs, Klemetti 1997 & Takala 1994 (N=195) showed no difference between group classes & control group for pain or sick leave at 1 or 6 months.

Revel 1994 – RCT; N=60; Individual sessions of exercises (incl. proprioceptive re-education – slow neck movements to follow moving target) relieved pain by 36% & improved functional status by 33% relative to waiting list controls.

Mechanical traction (Level II - CCT): Goldie 1970 – CCT; N=73; patient-assessed improvement in traction group relative to no treatment group; low quality (0/5). Zylbergold 1985, Lee 1996 & British Assoc. of Physical Medicine 1966 excluded.

Therapeutic ultrasound (Level I – RCT): Lee 1997 – RCT; N=26; myofascial trigger point neck pain; no difference in pain between ultrasound & placebo ultrasound. Other outcomes not assessed.

No evidence found: EMG biofeedback, massage, thermotherapy, electrical stimulation, TENS, & combined rehabilitation interventions. Persson 1997 also excluded.

There is scientific evidence to support and recommend use of proprioceptive & therapeutic exercises for chronic neck pain. There is a lack of evidence at present regarding whether to include or exclude use of thermotherapy, therapeutic massage, EMG biofeedback, mechanical traction, therapeutic ultrasound, TENS, electrical stimulation, & combined rehab interventions in daily practice of physical rehabilitation of patients with acute & chronic neck pain.

Reference	Patients	Interventions	Study designs
Gross et al, 2002a [140]	**Include:** mechanical neck disorders, neck disorders with headache of cervical origin, neck disorders with radicular signs and symptoms. **Exclude:** neck disorders with long tract signs, those caused by rheumatic or neurological diseases, fractures or dislocations, non-mehanical headache.	Manipulation, manipulation combined with mobilisation, manipulation combined with other modalities, manipulation combined with exercise (low-technology or high technology), multimodal care (manipulation & other manual therapies). Also harm from manipulation & mobilisation were studied.	Therapy question: RCT, quasi-RCT, higher quality systematic reviews. Harm question: RCT, quasi-RCT, surveys, higher quality systematic reviews.
Gross et al, 2002b [147]	**Include:** Working age (18–65 years) patients with neck or shoulder pain. **Exclude:** Patients with acute trauma, neoplasms, inflammatory or neurologic diseases. Studies of postoperative pain & osteoporosis.	**Include:** Studies of one or more types of patient education strategies including (but not limited to) individualized teaching (ergonomic advice, postural advice, pain management strategies), group teaching (neck school), independent study (audiovisiual tapes) and combinations of methods. **Exclude:** Studies involving surgery & injections excluded.	RCTs & CCTs

Outcomes	Search strategy	Results	Conclusions
Pain, disability/ function, patient satisfaction. Estimates of adverse event rate of minor (common & transient), moderate (reversible serious), major (irreversible serious) complications.	Medline, Embase, MANTIS, CINAHL, ICL, CCTR – to January 1998. Personal files of specialists, manual searches of published textbooks, reference tracking. Additional searches for harm: cohort studies and surveys on MEDLINE, CINAHL, EMBASE – to June 1997. Reference tracking and personal files – to January 1999.	Manipulation or mobilisation alone similar to placebo, wait period, control for pain relief. High-technology exercises superior to manipulation alone for decreasing long-term pain. Manipulation plus low technology exercises superior to manipulation alone for decreasing long-term pain. Manipulation plus low technology exercise superior to manipulation alone for patient satisfaction. Manipulation plus low-technology exercise superior to high technology exercise alone for patient satisfaction. Multi-modal care (including some manipulation/mobilisation/exercise) superior to control, other physical interventions & rest. Estimates for serious complications for manipulation (1 in 20,000 to 5 in 10,000,000).	Stronger evidence: a multi-modal management strategy using mobilisation or manipulation plus exercise relieves mechanical neck pain. Weaker evidence: either manipulation or mobilisation alone is less beneficial than when combined with exercise. The risk rate is uncertain.
Include: At least one outcome measure must have been used to measure response to treatment. Outcomes expected included pain, tenderness, range of motion, medication use, activities of daily living, return to work status, patient performance or costs of treatment. Primary outcome is pain.	Described in another review	271 patients (mean age 28.7 to 43 years) in 3 RCTs with 104 patients receiving patient education interventions. Mean (SD) duration of treatment = 44.3 (17.4) days & duration of follow-up from 21 days to 84 days. **Group Teaching (Neck School):** Kamwendo (1991) – 2 group teaching methods vs. no treatment for chronic neck disorders. No sig. reduction in pain reported (p>0.05). No treatment effect for traditional neck school + compliance measures (SMD at four weeks of treatment [morning] = -0.366 [95% CI: -0.951, 0.219]) or 4 hours traditional neck school alone (SMD at four weeks of treatment [morning] = 0.073 [95% CI: -0.513, 0.659]). Not clear if any patients advised not to seek additional information – confounding may be present. **Individualized Teaching (Advice):** Koes, 1992 - anti-inflammatories, analgesics and individualized patient education (advice) vs placebo in 25 patients with neck pain. Placebo was de-tuned diathermy and de-tuned ultrasound. SMD of 0.244 (95% CI: -0.577, 1.065) at 3 weeks, not sig., remained non-significant at later follow up. Not noted if physiotherapists give additional advice or patients advised not to seek additional information. McKinney (1989) compared two individualized teaching methods in acute whiplash.	Patient education utilising individualised or group instructional strategies has not been shown to be beneficial in reducing pain for mechanical neck disorders.

Reference	Patients	Interventions	Study designs
Gross et al, 2002c [149]	**Include:** Aged 18 or over with neck disorder grade 1 or 2. **Exclude:** Studies that include subjects with definite or possible neurological deficit; those with neck pain caused by other pathological entities (eg diffuse connective tissue diseases) & those with headache without mechanical neck disorders.	**Include:** Studies used one or more physical medicine modalities (incl. cervical orthoses, therapeutic heat or cold, traction, biofeedback, exercise, electrotherapy, phototherapies (laser therapy), & acupuncture. **Exclude:** Invasive therapies (injections or surgery)	RCT & CCT

At 4 weeks, individualized education for group 3 (demonstrated mobilization exercises, verbal and written instruction on posture correction, on the use of a collar, heat sources, muscle relaxation and analgesics) gave sig. pain relief compared to group 1 (general advice about mobilization after a 10 to 14 day period of rest and use of analgesics) (SMD = -0.617 [95% CI: -1.048, -0.186]). At 6 weeks of treatment no longer any sig. difference between groups (SMD = -0.371 [95% CI: -0.796, 0.054]). Co-intervention (patient seeking additional information about their problem) was not reported.
Number of trials using any one educational variable too few to make any conclusive statement of benefit, no benefit or harm in terms of reducing pain.

Any outcomes included to measure response to treatment – primary outcome used was pain.

Sources: Medlars, Embase, Chirolars, Index to chiropractic literature, CINAHL; searched 1985 to Dec 1993.
National Technical Information Services & Conference Proceedings Index searched for unpublished data. Science Citation Index searched. Reference lists of articles found & Science Citation Index used to track key references. Known authors, content experts, professions of chiropractic, education, medicine & physical therapy, national & international agencies, foundations & associations contacted for funded, published or unpublished research.

Quality: 5 high scores, 6 moderately high & 2 weak studies. Mean score 3.5, median 3.
Spray & Stretch: 1 RCT, no sig. difference between active & placebo (SMD= 0.101 (95% CI –0.597, 0.799)) or control group (– 0.299 (95%CI –0.940, 0.341) p>0.05). Low statistical power.
Laser therapy: 3 RCTs. Thorsen 1992, median effect size VAS-function at 2 weeks is 3.36 (95%CI 0.62, 2.38) Thorsen 1991, median effect size function is 0.80 (95%CI –4.07, 9.67). Combined p-values for subacute & chronic neck disorders, 2-tailed p-value=0.1988, chronic neck pain only 2-tailed p-value=0.6287. Treatment with laser not sig. reduce pain compared to control treatment, low power to detect.
Electromagnetic therapy: 2 RCTs Foley-Nolan, 1992; acute neck pain – 4 weeks, p=0.05.
Foley-Nolan, 1990; chronic neck pain – 3 weeks, p=0.02 – Combined 2 p-values=0.0089. No sig. changes at 6 & 12 weeks.
Infra-red light: 1 placebo-controlled trial (Lewith 1981); chronic neck pain; Non-sig. treatment effect reported (chi-square=3.28; p=0.07). Not enough statistical power.
Acupuncture: 2 RCTs. Petrie, 1983; chronic neck pain; acupuncture vs. placebo; positive treatment effect p<0.01. Loy, 1983; chronicity not specified; 87.2% improvement in 6 weeks of treatment in electroacupuncture group & 53.9% in

Reference	Patients	Interventions	Study designs
Smith et al, 2000 [153]	Patients with neck or back pain	**Include:** Acupuncture with or without electrical stimulation, or laser acupuncture, compared with an inactive control group. **Exclude:** Comparisons with other active treatments.	RCTs with group size >=10.

traction with shortwave diathermy group.
Traction: 3 RCTs. Goldie, 1970; controlled trial; traction vs. analgesics, muscle relaxants & postural advice. Difference very small, no statistical analysis reported. Pennie ,1990; no sig. treatment effect reported between traction, exercise & education vs. collar and exercise. Loy, 1983, as for acupuncture.
Exercise: Goldie, 1970; as for traction. Levoska 1993; active muscle training vs. passive stretching plus heat & massage; Sig. difference for active exercise (p<0.05 at 5 treatments & p<0.01 at 3 months or 1 year follow up).
TENS: Nordemar, 1981; TENS vs. collar, rest, education & analgesics; SMD=-0.549 (95%CI –1.492, 0.394), no sig. difference.

| Pain outcomes. | Sources & dates searched from & to: Medline (1966 to Aug 1998); Embase (1980 to Aug 1998); CINAHL (1982 to 1998); PsychLit (1982 to 1998); Pubmed (1998); The Cochrane Library (Issue 3, 1998); Oxford Pain Relief Database (1950 to 1994). Keywords used: Free-text search using all variants of term 'acupuncture' & 'electroacupuncture' with 'back*', 'lumb*', 'sciatica', 'myofasci*', 'radicul*', 'spondy*', 'neck*', 'cervic*', & 'whiplash' Reference lists searched. | Petrie & Hazleman (1986) compared 8 treatment sessions of acupuncture at 5 traditional points (20 mins, 2 times per week for 4 weeks) with sham TENS in chronic neck pain. No sig. differences in pain at 1 week and 21-28 days post-treatment. NNT=280 for acupuncture due to <50% success rate. (Oxford Pain Validity Scale=7/16).
Coan (1981) compared minimum 10 treatment sessions of traditional classical oriental meridian acupuncture, with or without electrical stimulation 3 or 4 times per week with a delayed treatment control group, who had no intervention/contact. After 12 weeks, 12/15 improve on acupuncture vs. 2/15 on control, relative benefit 6.0 (95%CI 1.6 to 22) – 'improved' not defined. (OPVS=5/16). | | OPVS useful tool for assessing validity in qualitative reviews. With acupuncture for chronic back and neck pain, we found most valid trials tended to be negative. There is no convincing evidence for the analgesic efficacy of acupuncture for back or neck pain. |

Reference	Patients	Interventions	Study designs
Karjalainen et al, 2003a [145]	Patients with subacute back pain (> 4 weeks < 3 months)	Multidisciplinary biopsychosocial rehabilitation for working age patients.	RCTs, CCTs
Karjalainen et al, 2003b [155]	**Include:** Working age (18–65 years) patients with neck or shoulder pain. **Exclude:** Patients with acute trauma, neoplasms, inflammatory or neurologic diseases. Studies of postoperative pain & osteoporosis.	**Include:** Multidisciplinary in-patient or out-patient rehab program – i.e. physician's consultation plus psychological, social or vocational intervention or combination. **Exclude:** Interventions consisting of medical treatment and physiotherapy only. Neck schools included in different review.	RCT & CCT

Outcomes	Search strategy	Results	Conclusions
Pain intensity, global status, disorder specific functional status, generic functional status or quality of life, ability to work, health care consumption and costs, patient satisfaction.	MEDLINE, EMBASE, PsycLIT, CENTRAL, Medic, the Science Citation Index, reference checking and consulting experts in the rehabilitation field – to November 2002 for EMBASE & MEDLINE.	**Quality of included studies:** Lindstrom (1992) 4/10, no blinding. Loisel (1997) 2/10, inadequate randomisation, no blinding, unclear baseline characteristics. Multidisciplinary rehabilitation that includes a work place visit or an occupational health care intervention helps patients return to work faster, results in less sick leave, decreases subjective disability.	This evidence is based on only 2 relevant trials & both had methodological shortcomings.
Pain intensity; global status; disorder specific functional status; generic functional status or quality of life; ability to work; health care consumption & costs; satisfaction with treatment.	Sources: Medline (1966 to April 1998); PsychLIT (1967 to April 1998); Embase (1988 to April 1998); The Cochrane Library; Medic (Finnish medical database); Science Citation Index. Full search strategy given in paper. Reference lists screened; 24 experts in field of rehab consulted.	**Quality:** Jensen, 1995 - 3/10; Patient characteristics not described adequately; method of randomisation not described. Ekberg, 1994 - 2/10; Non-randomised allocation. Both studies – blinding of patients but not described for therapists; baseline characteristics differed between groups; co-interventions not avoided; intention-to-treat not used. Overall no fatal methodological flaws, although info missing on some methodological quality items. Ekberg, 1994 – 1) active multidisciplinary rehabilitation (n=53) for 8 wks, 2 hours a day, 4 days per wk (incl. physical training, info, education, social interaction, & work place visit) vs. 2) traditional treatment (n=40) (incl. physiotherapy, medication, rest, & sick leave). Dropouts: 14 (13%) at 2 years. Pain (10-pt VAS): baseline 1) 6.1, 2) 6.0; at 12 mths 1) 5.3, 2) 5.4; at 24 mths 1) 5.0, 2) 4.8. General functional status: numerical data not reported. Sick leave (days/yr): baseline 1) 28, 2) 25; at 12 mths 1) 14, 2) 22; at 24 mths 1) 12, 2) 14. Jensen, 1995 – 1) 5 wks in-patient multimodal cognitive-behavioural treatment (n=29). Behavioural component by psychologist direct to patient vs. 2) psychologist as coach to other health professionals (n=37). Dropouts: 4 (6%) at 6 mths. Pain (100mm VAS): baseline 1) 52.2, 2) 51.6; after rehab 1) 45.0, 2)42.4; at 6 mths 1)45.2, 2) 48.5. Disorder specific functional status (HAQ): baseline 1) 27.1, 2) 24.1; after rehab 1) 30.1, 2) 27.0; at 6 mths 1) 26.2, 2) 25.6. Days off in 6 mths: baseline 1) 138, 2) 140; at 12 mths 1) 110, 2) 105; at 18 mths 1) 90, 2) 90.	There appears to be little scientific evidence for the effectiveness of multidisciplinary biopsychosocial rehab compared with other rehab facilities on neck & shoulder pain. Multidisciplinary rehab is a commonly used intervention for chronic neck & shoulder complaints, therefore we see an urgent need for high quality trials in this field.

Reference	Patients	Interventions	Study designs
Kjellman et al, 1999 [141]	Patients with on-going neck pain.	Physiotherapy or chiropractic treatment modalities.	**Include:** RCTs only, written in English or Scandinavian language. **Exclude:** Studies involving back and neck pain.
Van der Heijden et al [148]	Patients with back or neck pain.	Traction technique included in treatment regimen.	**Include:** Random allocation **Exclude:** Abstracts, unpublished studies, alternate treatment allocation.

Outcomes	Search strategy	Results	Conclusions
None given	Medline & Cinahl (1966 to 1995). Keywords used: 'randomised' used with free-text words, such as neck, cervical, pain, physiotherapy, physical therapy, chiropractic, exercise, rehabilitation, studies, outcomes, and evaluation. Reference lists searched.	**Quality of included studies:** 9 of 27 had quality score (QS) >=50 (range 24 to 62). Worst section was in measurement of effect (patient blinded or time restriction, relevant outcome measures and blinded outcome assessment) and intervention (avoiding simultaneous treatments & comparison with placebo). Also low scores for adequate randomisation, comparable baseline characteristics & comparisons with an existing treatment modality. Small sample sizes. **Effectiveness of interventions:** Acute: 4 studies, positive outcomes in 3. 1 with QS >=50 – electromagnetic therapy. Chronic: 12 studies, 9 positive outcomes. 2 with QS >=50 of manipulation and electromagnetic therapy. 3 equivalent/negative outcomes – 2 with QS >=50 of traction & acupuncture. Mixed: 11 studies. 6 positive. 3 with QS >=50 of electromagnetic therapy, manipulation & active physiotherapy treatment, 5 equivalent/negative outcomes – 1 with QS >=50. 6 of 9 studies with QS>=50 had positive outcomes – 1 active physio (Levoska, 1993), 3 electromagnetic therapy (Foley-Nolan, 1992; Foley-Nolan, 1990; Trock, 1994), & 2 manipulation (Boline, 1995; Cassidy, 1992). Equivalent/negative outcomes in 3 studies with QS>=50. 1 acupuncture (Petrie, 1986) & 2 cervical traction (British Assoc of Physical Medicine, 1966; Klaber Moffett, 1990).	Our analyses demonstrate that few randomised clinical trials on neck problems are of high methodological quality and comprise a sufficiently long follow up time. In the studies that did show higher quality, three different interventions led to a slight tendency towards positive results, but the number of publications considered was inadequate to allow general conclusions to be drawn.
Clinically relevant outcome measures: global estimate of improvement, pain, mobility, functional status.	Sources: Medline (1966 to 1992), Embase (1974 to 1992), Index to Chiropractic Literature (1980 to 1992), Physiotherapy Index (1986 to 1992). Keywords: Medline: traction, therapeutic use, not fractures, musculoskeletal diseases, joint diseases, spinal	**Quality:** 3 studies of neck pain; 1 scored over 50 points. Goldie & Landquist; chronic cervical pain & brachialgia; i) intermittent motorised traction (n=26) vs. ii) isometric exercises (n=24) vs. iii) no intervention (n=23). Patient global estimate of improvement at 3 weeks: i) 17/26 improved vs. ii) 17/24 vs. iii) 7/23. British Association of Physical Medicine; cervical pain; i) continuous motorised traction, hot packs & mobilising exercises (n=114) vs. ii) sham traction (positioning exercises) (n=114) vs. iii) collar (n=120) vs. iv) placebo (de-tuned, ultrashort waves)	The available RCTs do not allow conclusions about effectivenes of cervical or lumbar traction. Therefore, intervention studies do not support common practical recommendations or clinical guidelines about traction mainly based on rationale of spinal elongation.

Reference	Patients	Interventions	Study designs
White et al, 1999 [146]	**Include:** Patients with neck pain – also studies including subjects with either neck or back pain, but not both. **Exclude:** Patients with headache & those with pain in multiple sites.	**Include:** Acupuncture versus control procedure. Includes needle acupuncture, electroacupuncture and laser acupuncture. **Exclude:** Comparisons of 2 different types of acupuncture.	RCTs only

Outcomes	Search strategy	Results	Conclusions
	diseases, neck, backache, cervical, adverse effects, comparative studies, evaluation studies, outcome & process assessment, physical therapy, epidemiology, statistics, science.	(n=66) vs. v) placebo (analgesics) (n=52). Patient global estimate of improvement at 4 weeks: i) 24/114 improved; ii) 26/114; iii) 29/120; iv) 14/66; & v) 8/52. Zylbergold & Piper; subacute cervical pain; i) continuous motorised traction (25lbs, hot packs, neck school, mobilising & isometric exercises) (n=25) vs. intermittent motorised traction (25lbs, hot packs, neck school, mobilising & isometric exercises) (n=25) vs. manual traction (hot packs, neck school, mobilising & isometric exercises) (n=25) vs. hot packs, neck school, mobilising & isometric exercises (n=25).	
Not specified	Sources & dates searched from & to: Search date: January 1998 Medline (1966 to 1997); Embase (1974 to 1997); The Cochrane Library (Issue 1, 1998); & CISCOM (December 1997) (complementary medicine database). Keywords used: neck pain, cervical, cervicogenic, osteoarthritis, acupuncture & controlled trial. Reference lists searched.	Quality of included studies: 18 studies excluded. Max. score 4/5, only 1 study, 6 studies had 3/5. Needle acupuncture: 12 studies. Results balanced between positive & negative – 8 with quality 3 or above, 5 negative & 3 positive for acupuncture. Acupuncture superior to waiting list in one study. [Coan et al, 1982] 3 studies compared acupuncture with existing physio – groups equal in 2 studies [David et al, 1998; Kisiel & Lindh, 1996] & acupuncture superior in 1 study [Loy, 1983]. Needle acupuncture compared with indistinguishable controls in five studies [Emery & Lythgoe, 1986; Gallacchi et al, 1981; Junnila, 1982; Lundeberg et al, 1991; Thomas et al, 1991]. All but one [Junnila, 1982] produced negative results. Laser acupuncture better than sham laser in 2 studies [Ceccherelli et al, 1989; Kreczi & Klinger, 1986] & no different in 1 study [Gallacchi et al, 1981]. 3 studies looked at short-term pain relief: acupuncture superior to sham laser [Irnich et al, 2001], but not superior to an indistinguishable sham acupuncture [Lundeberg et al, 1991; Thomas et al, 1991].	Hypothesis that acupuncture efficacious in treatment of neck pain not supported by the evidence from controlled trials. More, better designed trials of acupuncture required before can be used in management of neck pain.

Table 3 Evidence table of systematic reviews on WAD, which were used to identify relevant individual studies

Reference	Patients	Interventions	Study designs
McClune et al, 2002 [12]	**Include:** All aspects of WAD including clinical and non-clinical studies on Quebec Task Force (QTF) grades 0-III. **Exclude:** QTF grade IV i.e. fracture or dislocation & surgical interventions.	Patients' informational needs	Clinical and non clinical articles encompassing the wide range of patients' informational needs.
Scholten-Peeters, 2002 [6]	**Include:** Patients with whiplash grade I (neck pain, stiffness or tenderness only with no physical signs) or grade II (neck symptoms & musculoskeletal signs). **Exclude:** studies including patients other than those with whiplash.	Physiotherapy interventions	**Include:** Systematic reviews, randomised clinical/controlled trials & prospective studies. **Exclude:** Not English, French, German or Dutch.

Outcomes	Search strategy	Results	Conclusions & comments
Good recovery, return to normal activity, reduction of chronicity.	Reports from the Quebec Task Force & the British Columbia Whiplash Initiative. Medline & psycINFO 1994 – Oct 2001. Keywords: including whiplash, neck pain, treatment, biomechanics, education. Internet searches, personal database searches & citation tracking.	The main messages emerging were: • serious physical injury is rare • reassurance about good prognosis is important • over-medicalisation is detrimental • recovery is improved by early return to normal pre-accident activities, self-exercise, manual therapy • positive attitudes and beliefs are helpful in regaining activity levels • collars, rest, negative attitudes & beliefs delay recovery and contribute to chronicity.	The scientific evidence on WAD was robust and consistent enough to guide patient advice. Findings were synthesised into patient centred messages with the potential to reduce the risk of chronicity i.e. in *The Whiplash Book*.
Related to functions, activities or participation within scope of current physiotherapy practice.	Medline (1966 to June 2000); Cinahl (1982 to June 2000); Cochrane Controlled Trials Register & Cochrane Database of Systematic Reviews (Issue 3 2001); Database of the Dutch Institute of Allied Health Professions (1987 to June 2000). Keywords: including whiplash, neck sprain & neck injury, physiotherapy, physical therapy, behavioural therapy, education, massage, mobilization, exercises, & electrotherapy. References searched.	Peeters SR – 3 studies of acceptable validity concluded that rest may not be advised & active interventions tend to be more effective for whiplash. Magee SR – 8 studies of weak methodological quality reported a modest trend for positive effects of exercises, manual therapy & educational advice on posture for whiplash. Also evidence for ineffectiveness of rest & use of soft collar. Quebec Task Force SR – found weak evidence to limit immobilisation & to support manual mobilisation combined with other physiotherapy. Suggested mobilisations, exercises & advice on posture as adjunct to strategies promoting increased activity. More recent RCT confirms early return to usual activities preferable to rest & wearing soft collar. Case series found to address efficacy of physiotherapy for chronic whiplash. By consensus, agreed chronic whiplash like other chronic pain conditions. For chronic back pain, neck pain & fibromyalgia, 12 SRs indicate exercise, multidisciplinary treatments & behavioural therapies favourable in managing chronic pain, particularly in returning to normal activities & work.	Evidence for positive effect of active interventions, including exercise therapy, education, training functions & activities for acute whiplash. Chronic whiplash similar to other chronic pain conditions and evidence suggests advice, exercise therapy & education using behavioural principles.

Reference	Patients	Interventions	Study designs
Verhagen et al, 2002[13]	Patients suffering from grade I or II whiplash injury – neck complaints with or without musculoskeletal signs.	Any non-invasive, non-surgical or non-pharmacological treatment.	Include: Only RCTs or Controlled Clinical trials. Quality measured by overall methodolgical quality score, internal validity score & Delphi quality score. Scores compared. 'Acceptable validity' considered >50% of max. scores on at least 2 of 3 quality scales.
Binder, 2002[14]	Patients with acute or chronic whiplash.	Any treatments.	Systematic reviews (SRs) and RCTs only.

Outcomes	Search strategy	Results	Conclusions & comments
Main outcomes: pain, global perceived effect or participation in daily activities. Other outcomes included: well-being or disability.	Medline (1966 to June 1998), Cinahl (1982 to June 1998), Embase & PsychLit (1988 to June 1998), database of Dutch Institute of Allied Health Professions (1987 to August 1998) & Cochrane Controlled Trial Register. Reference lists checked.	11 studies reviewed, 8 'unacceptable validity'& 3 'acceptable validity'. **Active vs inactive or passive:** 2 'acceptable' studies. Exercise+ psychological education improved pain, global perceived effect & return to work more than TENS or ultrasound within 30 days. 'Act as usual' improved pain & stiffness initiated in 14 days, more than soft collar & sick leave. 3 'unacceptable' studies found sig. short-term improvements in pain with exercise therapy versus rest & soft collar & 1 found sig. benefit in control group too. **Active vs other active:** 1 low quality study showed 'phasic exercises' significantly greater effect on function than standard rehab exercises. **Inactive vs placebo:** 1 'acceptable' study reported PEMT within 72 hrs sig. better than placebo on pain & perceived global effect at 2 & 4 weeks but not 12 weeks – differences at baseline. **Conservative vs no treatment:** 4 low quality studies: 1 had no comparison between groups; 1 found no difference in pain & recovery between soft collar and no treatment; 2 studies found short-term but no long-term differences between no treatment groups and active intervention or ultra-reiz current.	**Author's conclusions:** Cautiously say 'rest makes rusty', active interventions (advice to stay active) may be effective in whiplash patients. Advising rest or immobilisation with collar not recommended. No recommendations can be made on the efficacy of treatments in chronic whiplash. Methodological quality low and paucity of chronic Whiplash studies. **Quality of paper:** Well-conducted SR of RCTs, not a great deal of detail in the results- possibly elsewhere in tables.
Pain; range of movement; function; adverse effects of treatment; return to work; level of disability (Neck Disability Index).	Usual Clinical Evidence search strategy (Medline, Embase, Cinahl, etc). Also searched Chirolars (Mantis) (1966 to Nov 1999), Bioethics (1973 to 1997) & Current Contents (1994 to 1997).	**Acute:** 4 SRs and 3 subsequent RCTs, 1 RCT in 2 SRs; PEMT sig. reduced pain after 4 weeks (p<0.05) vs. placebo PEMT, not sig. 3 months 1 SR found early mobilisation sig. increased pain relief & ROM after 4 & 8 weeks (p<0.01). 1 RCT found no sig. difference between early mobilisation vs. immobilisation at 12 weeks. 1 RCT found active mobilisation sig. improved symptoms started immediately after injury vs. rest plus collar (P<0.001) – 2 week delay not sig. 1 RCT in 1 SR found 'act as usual' plus NSAIDs improved subjective symptoms after 6 months vs. immobilisation plus 2 weeks sick leave, no sig. difference in objective ROM or sick leave taken & no difference in severe symptoms after 6 months (11% 'act as usual' vs. 15% immob. RR 0.75, 95%CI 0.08 to 1.42).	SRs and subsequent RCTs found limited evidence that electromagnetic field treatment versus placebo, early mobilisation versus immobilisation or rest plus collar, and multimodal treatment versus physical treatment significantly reduce pain, and that advice to act as usual plus anti-inflammatory drugs versus immobilisation plus

Reference	Patients	Interventions	Study designs
Magee et al, 2000 [15]	**Include:** male or female participants with sufficient soft tissue trauma to the cervical spine. **Exclude:** animal studies; people with rheumatic diseases, neurological/autonomic deficit & fractures.	Physical therapy intervention or programme within scope of physical therapy practice in Canada.	Prospective studies with control group or before-after study. Used 'Relevance' tool – Haywood & Dobbins. Systematic Overview Project. Edmonton: Alberta Heritage Foundation for Medical Research, 1997 – to see if met inclusion/exclusion criteria. Rated as 'strong', 'moderate' or 'weak' depending on the number of criteria with 'pass', 'moderate' or 'fail' assigned to them. Used critical appraisal tool to extract data from included studies – no ref.

Outcomes	Search strategy	Results	Conclusions & comments
		1 RCT found no sig. difference between regular exercise regimen & instructions to perform extra isometric exercise 3 x per day in pain or disability after 3 or 6 months. 1 RCT in 1 SR found that multimodal treatment (postural training, psychological support, eye fixation exercises, & manual treatment) sig. reduced pain vs. physical treatment (electrical, sonic, ultrasound & TENS) at end of treatment & at 1 & 6 months ($p<0.001$) and reduced time to return to work. **Chronic:** 1 SR found no physiotherapy trials.	14 days sick leave improves mild subjective symptoms. One RCT found no significant difference between different home exercise programmes versus each other in pain or disability.
Range of motion; pain; patient satisfaction.	Medline (1985-Feb 1997); CINAHL (1985-Dec 1996); EMBASE (1988-Dec 1996); Current Contents (1966-Mar 1997); HealthStar (1985-Dec 1996); Canadian Research Index (1982-1997); AMED (1985-1997); Chirolars (1990-1997); Agency for Health Care Policy & Research (AHCPR); & The Cochrane Library (1985-1997). Handsearched: Spine; Journal of Orthopedic and Sports Physical Therapy; Journal of Manipulatve Therapeutics from 1996 & 1997. References checked.	More than 11 different combinations of interventions; could not tell which particular treatment or combination more effective. 7 of 8 studies indicated improvement in treatment group, no study showed harmful effects of physical therapy. Positive trend highlighted by poor response of rest/analgesia group without physical therapy in McKinney's study, which had to be discontinued. In Foley-Nolan & Gennis studies subjects who had poor response to allocated intervention sought additional or alternative physical therapy. Positive trend in acute whiplash from exercise, manual therapy, pulsed electromagnetic therapy & educational advice on posture and positioning. Chronic injuries responded positively to holistic acupuncture in Su & Su's study. Soft collar use for 1–3 weeks not supported by evidence.	Exercises, manual therapy, educational advice on posture & pulsed electromagnetic therapy appear to have a positive effect on acute traumatic neck injuries following automobile accident. Evidence indicating acupuncture may be useful in chronic whiplash. Evidence that use of soft cervical collars used alone of no value in treating acute injuries although subjects felt more comfortable.

Reference	Patients	Interventions	Study designs
Spitzer et al, 1995 [2]	**Include:** acceleration deceleration injury to the neck from a motor vehicle collision. **Exclude:** minimal (grade 0 injury), shaken baby syndrome & diving injury	A range of physiotherapy interventions: soft collars, rest, cervical pillow, manual mobilisation, exercise, traction, postural advice, passive modalities & electrotherapies, psychosocial interventions, prescribed function, acupuncture.	Data from many published & original studies over 2 decades. Only original research was considered as scientific.

Outcomes	Search strategy	Results	Conclusions & comments
Absence from usual activities, occurrence of a relapse, cost of the injury.	Broad search of Medline, TRIS, NTIS from 1980 to September 1994. Published and unpublished studies known to task force members. Agencies e.g. Insurance Institute for Highway Safety. Scanning of reference lists.	A series of recommendations were made i.e. encourage early return to usual activity, promote mobility; discourage soft collars; in the acute stage, treatments for pain relief, including manipulative treatments, might be beneficial with promotion of activity; reassurance of the likelihood of a good prognosis was important; dependence on health professionals and extensive use of manipulation should be discouraged.	The study found little scientifically rigorous information. Most conclusions were based on the best available evidence & consensus.

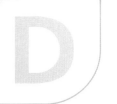

Appendix D

The CSP guidelines development group on whiplash associated disorder (WAD)

Helping us reach a consensus

Please read each statement carefully, decide the extent to which you agree or disagree with it and mark one box. However note that a few questions are open and require a few words rather than a tick. It would be helpful if you could return the form to us by 18th September 2003.

If you would like to make more detailed comments please use the reverse of this questionnaire. Ensure that you emphasise the question number that your comment refers to.

	Strongly agree	Agree	Neither agree nor disagree	Disagree	Strongly disagree	Don't know
Questions 1–4 cover general considerations concerning WAD						
1 The following indicate increased likelihood of severe symptoms						
a. Looking to one side during a rear-end collision	☐	☐	☐	☐	☐	☐
b. Poorly positioned headrest	☐	☐	☐	☐	☐	☐
2 These pre-existing factors indicate that a poor prognosis is likely following WAD						
a. Pre-existing degenerative changes	☐	☐	☐	☐	☐	☐
b. Pre-trauma headaches	☐	☐	☐	☐	☐	☐
c. Pre-trauma neck ache	☐	☐	☐	☐	☐	☐
d. Low level of job satisfaction	☐	☐	☐	☐	☐	☐
e. Injury occurring at 50 years of age and above	☐	☐	☐	☐	☐	☐
f. Being female	☐	☐	☐	☐	☐	☐
3 The following post-injury factors suggest that a poor prognosis is likely following WAD						
a. Headache for more than six months following injury	☐	☐	☐	☐	☐	☐
b. Neurological signs present after injury	☐	☐	☐	☐	☐	☐
c. Unresolved legal issues	☐	☐	☐	☐	☐	☐
4 The natural history of WAD suggests that						
a. It is good practice for physiotherapists to advise people with WAD that they are very likely to recover	☐	☐	☐	☐	☐	☐

	Strongly agree	Agree	Neither agree nor disagree	Disagree	Strongly disagree	Don't know

Questions 5–12 consider the examination and assessment strategies of people with WAD

5   In the acute stage, entering physiotherapy services is best prioritised by:

	Strongly agree	Agree	Neither agree nor disagree	Disagree	Strongly disagree	Don't know
a. A physiotherapist working in the Accident and Emergency department	☐	☐	☐	☐	☐	☐
b. A physiotherapist assessing individual people by telephone	☐	☐	☐	☐	☐	☐
c. A physiotherapist screening individual people using the information provided on the referral form	☐	☐	☐	☐	☐	☐
d. A physiotherapist screening individual people	☐	☐	☐	☐	☐	☐

6   The following factors make an individual person a higher priority at the assessment/screening stage

	Strongly agree	Agree	Neither agree nor disagree	Disagree	Strongly disagree	Don't know
a. The injury occurred more recently	☐	☐	☐	☐	☐	☐
b. The symptoms have been present over a longer time period	☐	☐	☐	☐	☐	☐
c. Person's activities of daily living are disrupted	☐	☐	☐	☐	☐	☐
d. Person is off work	☐	☐	☐	☐	☐	☐

7   A physiotherapist should always test for instability when a person with WAD has one or more of the following:

	Strongly agree	Agree	Neither agree nor disagree	Disagree	Strongly disagree	Don't know
a. Inability to support his/her head	☐	☐	☐	☐	☐	☐
b. Dysphagia	☐	☐	☐	☐	☐	☐
c. Tongue paraesthesia	☐	☐	☐	☐	☐	☐
d. A metallic taste in his/her mouth	☐	☐	☐	☐	☐	☐
e. Facial lip paraesthesia	☐	☐	☐	☐	☐	☐
f. Bilateral limb paraesthesia	☐	☐	☐	☐	☐	☐
g. Quadrilateral limb paraesthesia	☐	☐	☐	☐	☐	☐
h. Nystagmus	☐	☐	☐	☐	☐	☐

8   Instability is tested by the following methods:

	Strongly agree	Agree	Neither agree nor disagree	Disagree	Strongly disagree	Don't know
a. Distraction tests	☐	☐	☐	☐	☐	☐
b. Sagittal stress tests	☐	☐	☐	☐	☐	☐
c. The Sharp-Purser sagittal stress test	☐	☐	☐	☐	☐	☐
d. Coronal stress tests	☐	☐	☐	☐	☐	☐
e. Alar ligament stress tests	☐	☐	☐	☐	☐	☐

9. Please list the textbook(s) that you would recommend for physiotherapists for details of assessing patients WAD?

	Strongly agree	Agree	Neither agree nor disagree	Disagree	Strongly disagree	Don't know
10 Do these recognised barriers to recovery from chronic pain apply to people with WAD?						
a. High fear of pain and movement (fearing that pain and/or movement leads to harm)	☐	☐	☐	☐	☐	☐
b. High tendency to catastrophise (thinking the worst about the pain)	☐	☐	☐	☐	☐	☐
c. Low self-efficacy (lacking confidence in ability to undertake a particular activity)	☐	☐	☐	☐	☐	☐
d. Severe anxiety	☐	☐	☐	☐	☐	☐
e. Evidence of severe depression	☐	☐	☐	☐	☐	☐
f. Low pain locus of control (believing that it is impossible to control the pain)	☐	☐	☐	☐	☐	☐
g. High use of passive coping strategies (withdrawal/passing on responsibility for pain control to others)	☐	☐	☐	☐	☐	☐
h. Series of previously failed treatments	☐	☐	☐	☐	☐	☐
i. Person currently off work as a result of the pain	☐	☐	☐	☐	☐	☐
j. Chronic widespread pain	☐	☐	☐	☐	☐	☐

k. Do you think that there are any other barriers to recovery for WAD sufferers? Please specify.

	Strongly agree	Agree	Neither agree nor disagree	Disagree	Strongly disagree	Don't know
11 The barriers to recovery should be assessed at the following stages after injury:						
a. Less than 2 weeks after injury	☐	☐	☐	☐	☐	☐
b. After 2 weeks and before 6 weeks	☐	☐	☐	☐	☐	☐
c. After 6 weeks and before 12 weeks	☐	☐	☐	☐	☐	☐
d. At 12 weeks or more	☐	☐	☐	☐	☐	☐
12 A major aim of physiotherapy treatment should be?						
a. To relieve symptoms	☐	☐	☐	☐	☐	☐
b. To improve function	☐	☐	☐	☐	☐	☐
c. To facilitate empowerment of the person	☐	☐	☐	☐	☐	☐
d. To get the person back to normal activity/work	☐	☐	☐	☐	☐	☐

	Strongly agree	Agree	Neither agree nor disagree	Disagree	Strongly disagree	Don't know

Questions 13–15 consider physiotherapeutic intervention in the first two weeks after injury

13 The following should be used to enhance the effect of rest and analgesia in reducing pain:

	Strongly agree	Agree	Neither agree nor disagree	Disagree	Strongly disagree	Don't know
a. Soft collars	☐	☐	☐	☐	☐	☐
b. Manual mobilisation	☐	☐	☐	☐	☐	☐
c. Active exercise	☐	☐	☐	☐	☐	☐
d. A general active exercise programme devised for people with WAD	☐	☐	☐	☐	☐	☐
e. An active exercise programme devised for each individual following assessment	☐	☐	☐	☐	☐	☐
f. Interferential therapy	☐	☐	☐	☐	☐	☐
g. Ultrasound treatment	☐	☐	☐	☐	☐	☐
h. Massage	☐	☐	☐	☐	☐	☐
i. Soft tissue techniques	☐	☐	☐	☐	☐	☐
j. TENS	☐	☐	☐	☐	☐	☐
k. Laser treatment	☐	☐	☐	☐	☐	☐
l. Infrared light	☐	☐	☐	☐	☐	☐
m. Traction	☐	☐	☐	☐	☐	☐
n. Acupuncture	☐	☐	☐	☐	☐	☐
o. Relaxation	☐	☐	☐	☐	☐	☐
p. Education about the origin of the pain	☐	☐	☐	☐	☐	☐
q. Advice about coping strategies	☐	☐	☐	☐	☐	☐

14 The effect of early manual mobilisation techniques versus initial rest and soft collar

	Strongly agree	Agree	Neither agree nor disagree	Disagree	Strongly disagree	Don't know
a. Early manual mobilising is more effective than rest and a soft collar in improving neck range of movement	☐	☐	☐	☐	☐	☐
b. Early manual mobilisation is more effective than initial rest in improving function	☐	☐	☐	☐	☐	☐

15 An early physiotherapy programme versus initial rest and an exercise routine

	Strongly agree	Agree	Neither agree nor disagree	Disagree	Strongly disagree	Don't know
a. Early physiotherapy 'as usual' is more effective than initial rest followed by an exercise routine in improving function	☐	☐	☐	☐	☐	☐

	Strongly agree	Agree	Neither agree nor disagree	Disagree	Strongly disagree	Don't know
Questions 16–18 consider the physiotherapeutic intervention after two weeks and before twelve weeks since injury						
16 Manipulation and manual mobilisation						
a. Manipulation alone reduces pain	☐	☐	☐	☐	☐	☐
b. Manual mobilisation alone reduces pain	☐	☐	☐	☐	☐	☐
c. Manual mobilisation is more effective than a combination of ice and TENS in reducing pain	☐	☐	☐	☐	☐	☐
d. Manual mobilisation is more effective than acupuncture in reducing pain	☐	☐	☐	☐	☐	☐
e. Manual mobilisation is more effective than a single manipulation in reducing pain	☐	☐	☐	☐	☐	☐
f. Combined manipulation and manual mobilisation reduces pain	☐	☐	☐	☐	☐	☐
g. Combined manipulation and manual mobilisation is effective in improving function	☐	☐	☐	☐	☐	☐
17 Adverse events resulting from cervical manipulation						
a. The risk of serious adverse events (e.g. vertebrobasilar accidents) from manipulation is low	☐	☐	☐	☐	☐	☐
b. Minor or moderate adverse events (e.g. headache or nausea) occur in around half of all patients receiving cervical manipulation	☐	☐	☐	☐	☐	☐
18 The effect of other interventions						
a. Acupuncture is effective in reducing neck pain	☐	☐	☐	☐	☐	☐
b. Soft collars are effective in reducing pain	☐	☐	☐	☐	☐	☐
c. Education is effective in improving neck function	☐	☐	☐	☐	☐	☐
d. Advice about coping strategies is effective in enabling patients to return to normal activities	☐	☐	☐	☐	☐	☐
e. Traction is effective in reducing neck pain	☐	☐	☐	☐	☐	☐
f. TENS is effective in reducing neck pain	☐	☐	☐	☐	☐	☐
g. Infrared light is effective in reducing neck pain	☐	☐	☐	☐	☐	☐
h. Laser treatment is effective in reducing neck pain	☐	☐	☐	☐	☐	☐
i. Interferential therapy is effective in reducing neck pain	☐	☐	☐	☐	☐	☐
j. Ultrasound treatment is effective in reducing neck pain	☐	☐	☐	☐	☐	☐

	Strongly agree	Agree	Neither agree nor disagree	Disagree	Strongly disagree	Don't know
k. Massage is effective in reducing neck pain	☐	☐	☐	☐	☐	☐
l. Soft tissue techniques are effective in reducing neck pain	☐	☐	☐	☐	☐	☐
m. Muscle retraining and deep neck flexor activity is effective in improving function	☐	☐	☐	☐	☐	☐
n. Phasic exercise (rapid eye-hand-neck movements) is effective in improving function	☐	☐	☐	☐	☐	☐

Questions 19–23 consider the physiotherapeutic intervention for chronic whiplash i.e. 12 weeks or more since injury

19 Manipulation and manual mobilisation

	Strongly agree	Agree	Neither agree nor disagree	Disagree	Strongly disagree	Don't know
a. Manual mobilisation reduces pain	☐	☐	☐	☐	☐	☐
b. Manipulation reduces pain	☐	☐	☐	☐	☐	☐
c. Manual mobilisation is as effective as ice in reducing pain	☐	☐	☐	☐	☐	☐
d. Manual mobilisation is more effective than a combination of ice and TENS in reducing pain	☐	☐	☐	☐	☐	☐
e. Manual mobilisation is more effective than acupuncture in reducing pain	☐	☐	☐	☐	☐	☐
f. Manual mobilisation is more effective than a single manipulation in reducing pain	☐	☐	☐	☐	☐	☐
g. Combined manipulation and manual mobilisation reduce pain	☐	☐	☐	☐	☐	☐
h. Combined manipulation and manual mobilisation is effective in improving function	☐	☐	☐	☐	☐	☐

20 Comparing manipulation and exercise combined with manipulation alone

	Strongly agree	Agree	Neither agree nor disagree	Disagree	Strongly disagree	Don't know
a. Manipulation and exercise is more effective than manipulation alone in reducing long term pain	☐	☐	☐	☐	☐	☐
b. Manipulation and exercise is more effective than manipulation alone in terms of patient satisfaction	☐	☐	☐	☐	☐	☐
c. Manipulation and exercise is more effective than manipulation alone in improving function	☐	☐	☐	☐	☐	☐

21 Exercise therapy

	Strongly agree	Agree	Neither agree nor disagree	Disagree	Strongly disagree	Don't know
a. Standard exercise (stretching, isometric, isokinetic) is more effective than phasic exercise (rapid eye-hand-neck movements) in improving function	☐	☐	☐	☐	☐	☐
b. Strengthening exercise is more effective than endurance training in reducing pain	☐	☐	☐	☐	☐	☐

	Strongly agree	Agree	Neither agree nor disagree	Disagree	Strongly disagree	Don't know
c. Strengthening exercise is more effective than endurance training in improving function	☐	☐	☐	☐	☐	☐
d. Strengthening exercise is more effective than body awareness training in reducing pain	☐	☐	☐	☐	☐	☐
e. Strengthening exercise is more effective than body awareness training in improving function	☐	☐	☐	☐	☐	☐
f. Strengthening exercise is more effective than passive physiotherapy in reducing pain	☐	☐	☐	☐	☐	☐
g. Strengthening exercise is more effective than passive physiotherapy in improving function	☐	☐	☐	☐	☐	☐
h. Group exercise is effective in improving function	☐	☐	☐	☐	☐	☐
i. Proprioceptive exercise improves neck function	☐	☐	☐	☐	☐	☐
j. Neck schools are effective in improving function	☐	☐	☐	☐	☐	☐
k. Extension retraction exercises are effective in improving neck function	☐	☐	☐	☐	☐	☐
l. Mobilising exercises are effective in reducing pain	☐	☐	☐	☐	☐	☐
m. Exercises based on individual patient assessment is more effective than a generalised exercise programme in improving function	☐	☐	☐	☐	☐	☐
n. Advice about coping strategies combined with exercise is more effective than exercise alone in returning to normal activity	☐	☐	☐	☐	☐	☐

22 Acupuncture

	Strongly agree	Agree	Neither agree nor disagree	Disagree	Strongly disagree	Don't know
a. Acupuncture is more effective than massage in reducing pain	☐	☐	☐	☐	☐	☐
b. Acupuncture is more effective than sham acupuncture in reducing pain	☐	☐	☐	☐	☐	☐

23 Multidisciplinary psychosocial rehabilitation

	Strongly agree	Agree	Neither agree nor disagree	Disagree	Strongly disagree	Don't know
a. Multidisciplinary rehabilitation is more effective than traditional rehabilitation (physiotherapy, rest, sick leave) in improving function	☐	☐	☐	☐	☐	☐

Question 24 considers outcome of physiotherapeutic intervention for WAD

24 The following outcome measures are likely to be most effective for assessing progress of people with WAD

	Strongly agree	Agree	Neither agree nor disagree	Disagree	Strongly disagree	Don't know
a. For pain: The visual analogue scale	☐	☐	☐	☐	☐	☐
b. For function: The neck disability index	☐	☐	☐	☐	☐	☐

	Strongly agree	Agree	Neither agree nor disagree	Disagree	Strongly disagree	Don't know
c. For return to usual activities: The physiotherapy specific functional scale	☐	☐	☐	☐	☐	☐
d. For a patient centred measure: Measure yourself medical outcome profile (MYMOP)	☐	☐	☐	☐	☐	☐
e. For fear of movement: The Tampa Scale for Kinesiophobia (TSK)	☐	☐	☐	☐	☐	☐
f. Are there other measures that you use and can recommend?	☐	☐	☐	☐	☐	☐

Question 25 is about you

a. What is your specialist area in physiotherapy?

b. How long (in years) have you specialised in this area?

c. Can you tell us approximately how many people with WAD you treat per year?

Please return your completed form either on paper or electronically by Thursday 18th September 2003 to:

Helen Whittaker
Learning and Development
The Chartered Society of Physiotherapy
14 Bedford Row
London WC1R 4ED

or to: whittakerh@csp.org.uk

Thank you very much for your help in producing the CSP whiplash guidelines.

Appendix E

The CSP guidelines development group on whiplash associated disorder (WAD)

Helping us reach a consensus – Second round

Thank you very much for your help with the Delphi questionnaire. For this second round the percentage of respondents who marked each box in the first round is indicated beside each statement. For clarity we have not shown decimal places but the result is that rows do not necessarily total 100%. Note that some statements are new to this round. Please consider each statement, decide on your response now and mark one box. It would be helpful if you could return the form to us by 3rd November 2003.

Questions 1–4 cover general considerations concerning WAD

	Strongly agree	Agree	Neither agree nor disagree	Disagree	Strongly disagree	Don't know
1 The following indicate increased likelihood of severe symptoms						
a. Looking to one side during a rear-end collision	28%	43%	23%	5%	0%	3%
b. Poorly positioned headrest	28%	51%	13%	5%	0%	3%
2 These pre-existing factors indicate that a poor prognosis is likely following WAD						
a. Pre-existing degenerative changes	30%	53%	8%	8%	0%	3%
b. Pre-trauma headaches	20%	35%	23%	13%	3%	8%
c. Pre-trauma neck ache	20%	50%	18%	10%	0%	3%
d. Low level of job satisfaction	23%	50%	15%	5%	0%	8%
e. Injury occurring at 50 years of age and above	10%	30%	38%	15%	0%	8%
f. Being female	5%	25%	30%	30%	3%	8%
3 The following post-injury factors suggest that a poor prognosis is likely following WAD						
a. Headache for more than six months following injury	28%	58%	5%	8%	0%	3%
b. Neurological signs present after injury	45%	45%	8%	3%	0%	0%
c. Unresolved legal issues	25%	50%	18%	5%	0%	3%

	Strongly agree	Agree	Neither agree nor disagree	Disagree	Strongly disagree	Don't know
4 The natural history of WAD suggests that						
a. It is good practice for physiotherapists to advise people with WAD that they are very likely recover	68%	30%	3%	0%	0%	0%

Questions 5–12 consider the examination and assessment strategies of people with WAD

	Strongly agree	Agree	Neither agree nor disagree	Disagree	Strongly disagree	Don't know
5 In the acute stage, entering physiotherapy services is best prioritised by:						
a. A physiotherapist working in the Accident and Emergency department	49%	36%	10%	5%	0%	0%
b. A physiotherapist assessing individual people by telephone	13%	49%	21%	18%	0%	0%
c. A physiotherapist screening individual people using the information provided on the referral form	3%	26%	38%	23%	10%	0%
d. A physiotherapist screening individual people	28%	48%	15%	10%	0%	0%
6 The following factors make an individual person a higher priority at the assessment/screening stage						
a. The injury occurred more recently	30%	58%	8%	5%	0%	0%
b. The symptoms have been present over a longer time period	8%	30%	38%	23%	3%	0%
c. Person's activities of daily living are disrupted	50%	48%	3%	0%	0%	0%
d. Person is off work	78%	18%	3%	3%	0%	0%
7 A physiotherapist should always test for instability when a person with WAD has one or more of the following:						
a. Inability to support his/her head	37%	29%	11%	3%	11%	11%
b. Dysphagia	42%	34%	5%	3%	5%	11%
c. Tongue paraesthesia	47%	32%	3%	3%	5%	11%
d. A metallic taste in his/her mouth	39%	29%	8%	5%	5%	13%

	Strongly agree	Agree	Neither agree nor disagree	Disagree	Strongly disagree	Don't know
e. Facial or lip paraesthesia	37%	37%	5%	3%	5%	13%
f. Bilateral limb paraesthesia	47%	21%	13%	3%	5%	11%
g. Quadrilateral limb paraesthesia	50%	18%	8%	5%	8%	11%
h. Nystagmus	39%	29%	11%	3%	8%	11%
i Gait disturbance	☐	☐	☐	☐	☐	☐

8 Instability is tested by the following methods:

	Strongly agree	Agree	Neither agree nor disagree	Disagree	Strongly disagree	Don't know
a. Distraction tests	19%	28%	6%	13%	6%	28%
b. Sagittal stress tests	16%	28%	9%	6%	6%	34%
c. The Sharp-Purser sagittal stress test	36%	27%	6%	0%	3%	27%
d. Coronal stress tests	16%	25%	13%	3%	6%	38%
e. Alar ligament stress tests	27%	45%	3%	0%	6%	18%

9 This textbook could be recommend to assist physiotherapists in assessing people with WAD?

	Strongly agree	Agree	Neither agree nor disagree	Disagree	Strongly disagree	Don't know
a. Maitland G, Hengeveld E, Banks K, English K (2001) Maitland's Vertebral Manipulation (6th ed.) Butterworth Heinmann, Oxford.	☐	☐	☐	☐	☐	☐
b. Boyling J, Palastangar N (1994) Grieves Modern Manual Therapy 2nd Edition, Churchill Livingstone, Edinburgh.	☐	☐	☐	☐	☐	☐
c. Grieve G P (1988) Common Vertebral Joint Problems Churchill Livingstone, Edinburgh.	☐	☐	☐	☐	☐	☐
d. Petty N, Moore A P (2001) Neuro Musculoskeletal Examination and Assessment: A Handbook for Therapists (2nd ed.) Churchill Livingstone, Edinburgh.	☐	☐	☐	☐	☐	☐
e. Main C, Spanswick CC (2000) Pain Management: an Interdisciplinary Approach Churchill Livingstone, Edinburgh.	☐	☐	☐	☐	☐	☐
f. Oliver J, Middleditch A (1991) Functional Anatomy of the Spine Butterworth Heinmann Oxford.	☐	☐	☐	☐	☐	☐
g. Strong J (2002) Pain a Textbook for Therapists Churchill Livingstone, Edinburgh.	☐	☐	☐	☐	☐	☐

	Strongly agree	Agree	Neither agree nor disagree	Disagree	Strongly disagree	Don't know
h. Grant R (Ed.) (1994) Physical Therapy of the Cervical and Thoracic Spine (2nd ed.) Churchill Livingstone, New York.	☐	☐	☐	☐	☐	☐
j. Gifford L (ed.) Topical Issues in Pain (series)	☐	☐	☐	☐	☐	☐

10 Do these recognised barriers to recovery from chronic pain apply to people with WAD?

	Strongly agree	Agree	Neither agree nor disagree	Disagree	Strongly disagree	Don't know
a. High fear of pain and movement (fearing that pain and/or movement leads to harm)	90%	8%	0%	0%	0%	3%
b. High tendency to catastrophise (thinking the worst about the pain)	85%	13%	0%	0%	0%	3%
c. Low self-efficacy (lacking confidence in ability to undertake a particular activity)	60%	33%	5%	0%	0%	3%
d. Severe anxiety	58%	40%	0%	0%	0%	3%
e. Evidence of severe depression	56%	33%	8%	0%	0%	3%
f. Low pain locus of control (believing that it is impossible to control the pain)	78%	18%	3%	0%	0%	3%
g. High use of passive coping strategies (withdrawal/passing on responsibility for pain control to others)	68%	28%	3%	0%	0%	3%
h. Series of previously failed treatments	53%	45%	0%	3%	0%	0%
i. Person currently off work as a result of the pain	38%	38%	18%	8%	0%	0%
j. Chronic widespread pain	53%	38%	5%	5%	0%	0%
k. Poor understanding of the healing mechanism	☐	☐	☐	☐	☐	☐
l. Non compliance with treatment and advice	☐	☐	☐	☐	☐	☐
m. Problems in relationships with others	☐	☐	☐	☐	☐	☐
n. Negative expectations of treatment	☐	☐	☐	☐	☐	☐
o. Unrealistic expectations of treatment	☐	☐	☐	☐	☐	☐
p. Failure of the physiotherapist to address an individual person's needs	☐	☐	☐	☐	☐	☐
q. Poor clinical reasoning by the physiotherapist	☐	☐	☐	☐	☐	☐

	Strongly agree	Agree	Neither agree nor disagree	Disagree	Strongly disagree	Don't know
11 The barriers to recovery should be assessed at the following stages after injury:						
a. Less than 2 weeks after injury	22%	35%	24%	19%	0%	0%
b. After 2 weeks and before 6 weeks	32%	50%	8%	11%	0%	0%
c. After 6 weeks and before 12 weeks	34%	45%	13%	3%	5%	0%
d. At 12 weeks or more	38%	28%	8%	18%	8%	0%
12 A major aim of physiotherapy treatment should be?						
a. To relieve symptoms	28%	55%	10%	8%	0%	0%
b. To improve function	70%	30%	0%	0%	0%	0%
c. To facilitate empowerment of the person	88%	13%	0%	0%	0%	0%
d. To get the person back to normal activity/work	90%	10%	0%	0%	0%	0%

Questions 13–15 consider physiotherapeutic intervention in the first two weeks after injury

	Strongly agree	Agree	Neither agree nor disagree	Disagree	Strongly disagree	Don't know
13. The following should be used to enhance the effect of rest and analgesia in reducing pain:						
a. Soft collars	8%	13%	20%	25%	35%	0%
b. Manual mobilisation	10%	33%	26%	21%	10%	0%
c. Active exercise	69%	23%	8%	0%	0%	0%
d. A general active exercise programme devised for people with WAD	28%	46%	15%	5%	5%	0%
e. An active exercise programme devised for each individual following assessment	50%	30%	18%	3%	0%	0%
f. Interferential therapy	0%	13%	33%	18%	38%	0%
g. Ultrasound treatment	0%	13%	28%	23%	38%	0%
h. Massage	3%	35%	28%	18%	18%	0%

	Strongly agree	Agree	Neither agree nor disagree	Disagree	Strongly disagree	Don't know
i. Soft tissue techniques	8%	35%	25%	15%	18%	0%
j. TENS	5%	50%	28%	10%	8%	0%
k. Laser treatment	0%	0%	30%	28%	40%	3%
l. Infrared light	0%	3%	30%	20%	48%	0%
m. Traction	0%	5%	15%	38%	40%	3%
n. Acupuncture	10%	35%	33%	8%	13%	3%
o. Relaxation	18%	50%	26%	3%	3%	0%
p. Education about the origin of the pain	69%	21%	8%	3%	0%	0%
q. Advice about coping strategies	75%	23%	3%	0%	0%	0%

14 The effect of early manual mobilisation techniques versus initial rest and soft collar

	Strongly agree	Agree	Neither agree nor disagree	Disagree	Strongly disagree	Don't know
a. Early manual mobilising is more effective than rest and a soft collar in improving neck range of movement	43%	33%	10%	13%	0%	3%
b. Early manual mobilisation is more effective than initial rest in improving function	28%	40%	20%	13%	0%	0%

15 An early physiotherapy programme versus initial rest and an exercise routine

	Strongly agree	Agree	Neither agree nor disagree	Disagree	Strongly disagree	Don't know
a. Early physiotherapy 'as usual' is more effective than initial rest followed by an exercise routine in improving function	28%	15%	18%	25%	3%	13%

Questions 16–18 consider the physiotherapeutic intervention after two weeks and before twelve weeks since injury

16 Manipulation and manual mobilisation

	Strongly agree	Agree	Neither agree nor disagree	Disagree	Strongly disagree	Don't know
a. Manipulation alone reduces pain	3%	13%	28%	25%	33%	0%
b. Manual mobilisation alone reduces pain	5%	20%	25%	25%	25%	0%
c. Manual mobilisation is more effective than a combination of ice and TENS in reducing pain	8%	25%	30%	23%	3%	13%

E

	Strongly agree	Agree	Neither agree nor disagree	Disagree	Strongly disagree	Don't know
d. Manual mobilisation is more effective than acupuncture in reducing pain	0%	15%	33%	30%	0%	23%
e. Manual mobilisation is more effective than a single manipulation in reducing pain	5%	36%	33%	18%	0%	8%
f. Combined manipulation and manual mobilisation reduces pain	0%	43%	35%	18%	0%	5%
g. Combined manipulation and manual mobilisation is effective in improving function	3%	40%	30%	23%	0%	5%

17 Adverse events resulting from cervical manipulation

	Strongly agree	Agree	Neither agree nor disagree	Disagree	Strongly disagree	Don't know
a. The risk of serious adverse events (e.g. vertebrobasilar accidents) from manipulation is low	20%	65%	5%	10%	0%	0%
b. Minor or moderate adverse events (e.g. headache or nausea) occur in around half of all patients receiving cervical manipulation	0%	25%	20%	25%	15%	15%

18 The effect of other interventions

	Strongly agree	Agree	Neither agree nor disagree	Disagree	Strongly disagree	Don't know
a. Acupuncture is effective in reducing neck pain	20%	38%	20%	10%	0%	13%
b. Soft collars are effective in reducing pain	0%	25%	20%	30%	25%	0%
c. Education is effective in improving neck function	33%	60%	8%	0%	0%	0%
d. Advice about coping strategies is effective in enabling patients to return to normal activities	58%	43%	0%	0%	0%	0%
e. Traction is effective in reducing neck pain	3%	23%	28%	20%	28%	0%
f. TENS is effective in reducing neck pain	5%	53%	30%	8%	5%	0%
g. Infrared light is effective in reducing neck pain	0%	10%	23%	25%	35%	8%
h. Laser treatment is effective in reducing neck pain	0%	3%	23%	33%	28%	15%

	Strongly agree	Agree	Neither agree nor disagree	Disagree	Strongly disagree	Don't know
i. Interferential therapy is effective in reducing neck pain	3%	23%	25%	23%	20%	8%
j. Ultrasound treatment is effective in reducing neck pain	0%	20%	23%	30%	23%	5%
k. Massage is effective in reducing neck pain	3%	48%	33%	10%	8%	0%
l. Soft tissue techniques are effective in reducing neck pain	5%	54%	15%	10%	10%	5%
m. Muscle retraining and deep neck flexor activity is effective in improving function	13%	70%	10%	5%	3%	0%
n. Phasic exercise (rapid eye-hand-neck movements) is effective in improving function	0%	15%	38%	10%	0%	38%

Questions 19–23 consider the physiotherapeutic intervention for chronic whiplash
i.e. 12 weeks or more since injury

19 Manipulation and manual mobilisation

	Strongly agree	Agree	Neither agree nor disagree	Disagree	Strongly disagree	Don't know
a. Manual mobilisation reduces pain	15%	51%	13%	15%	5%	0%
b. Manipulation reduces pain	13%	39%	11%	32%	5%	0%
c. Manual mobilisation is as effective as ice in reducing pain	13%	18%	38%	8%	8%	15%
d. Manual mobilisation is more effective than a combination of ice and TENS in reducing pain	18%	18%	21%	15%	5%	23%
e. Manual mobilisation is more effective than acupuncture in reducing pain	5%	13%	31%	23%	8%	21%
f. Manual mobilisation is more effective than a single manipulation in reducing pain	8%	21%	36%	21%	5%	10%
g. Combined manipulation and manual mobilisation reduce pain	8%	44%	23%	13%	5%	8%
h. Combined manipulation and manual mobilisation is effective in improving function	10%	41%	26%	13%	8%	3%

	Strongly agree	Agree	Neither agree nor disagree	Disagree	Strongly disagree	Don't know
20 Comparing manipulation and exercise combined with manipulation alone						
a. Manipulation and exercise is more effective than manipulation alone in reducing long term pain	33%	51%	3%	8%	0%	5%
b. Manipulation and exercise is more effective than manipulation alone in terms of patient satisfaction	28%	38%	15%	3%	0%	15%
c. Manipulation and exercise is more effective than manipulation alone in improving function	31%	56%	5%	5%	0%	3%
21 Exercise therapy						
a. Standard exercise (stretching, isometric, isokinetic) is more effective than phasic exercise (rapid eye-hand-neck movements) in improving function	16%	26%	16%	0%	0%	42%
b. Strengthening exercise is more effective than endurance training in reducing pain	0%	13%	46%	21%	3%	18%
c. Strengthening exercise is more effective than endurance training in improving function	0%	13%	44%	26%	3%	15%
d. Strengthening exercise is more effective than body awareness training in reducing pain	3%	5%	46%	28%	3%	15%
e. Strengthening exercise is more effective than body awareness training in improving function	3%	8%	41%	28%	5%	15%
f. Strengthening exercise is more effective than passive physiotherapy in reducing pain	18%	28%	31%	13%	0%	10%
g. Strengthening exercise is more effective than passive physiotherapy in improving function	18%	44%	21%	10%	0%	8%
h. Group exercise is effective in improving function	15%	36%	31%	13%	0%	5%
i. Proprioceptive exercise improves neck function	10%	59%	26%	3%	0%	3%
j. Neck schools are effective in improving function	5%	38%	32%	11%	0%	14%

	Strongly agree	Agree	Neither agree nor disagree	Disagree	Strongly disagree	Don't know
k. Extension retraction exercises are effective in improving neck function	8%	41%	32%	14%	3%	3%
l. Mobilising exercises are effective in reducing pain	8%	72%	13%	3%	3%	3%
m. Exercises based on individual patient assessment is more effective than a generalised exercise programme in improving function	30%	45%	8%	15%	0%	3%
n. Advice about coping strategies combined with exercise is more effective than exercise alone in returning to normal activity	70%	28%	0%	0%	0%	3%

22 Acupuncture

	Strongly agree	Agree	Neither agree nor disagree	Disagree	Strongly disagree	Don't know
a. Acupuncture is more effective than massage in reducing pain	15%	18%	33%	8%	0%	28%
b. Acupuncture is more effective than sham acupuncture in reducing pain	10%	23%	18%	10%	3%	38%

23 Multidisciplinary psychosocial rehabilitation

	Strongly agree	Agree	Neither agree nor disagree	Disagree	Strongly disagree	Don't know
a. Multidisciplinary rehabilitation is more effective than traditional rehabilitation (physiotherapy, rest, sick leave) in improving function	28%	38%	18%	8%	0%	10%

Question 24 considers outcome of physiotherapeutic intervention for WAD

24 The following outcome measures are likely to be most effective for assessing progress of people with WAD

	Strongly agree	Agree	Neither agree nor disagree	Disagree	Strongly disagree	Don't know
a. For pain: The visual analogue scale	30%	55%	8%	5%	3%	0%
b. For function: The neck disability index	25%	45%	8%	0%	0%	23%
c. For return to usual activities: The physiotherapy specific functional scale	8%	35%	25%	0%	0%	33%
d. For a patient centred measure: Measure yourself medical outcome profile (MYMOP)	5%	25%	23%	0%	0%	48%
e. For fear of movement: The Tampa Scale for Kinesiophobia (TSK)	13%	18%	13%	0%	0%	58%

	Strongly agree	Agree	Neither agree nor disagree	Disagree	Strongly disagree	Don't know
f. For quality of life: SF-36	☐	☐	☐	☐	☐	☐
g. For patient satisfaction: The CSPs Clinical Audit tool, The patient feedback questionnaire	☐	☐	☐	☐	☐	☐
h. For anxiety and depression: The hospital anxiety and depression questionnaire	☐	☐	☐	☐	☐	☐
i. For self-efficacy: The Chronic Pain Self-Efficacy Scale (CPSES)	☐	☐	☐	☐	☐	☐

Please return your completed form either on paper or electronically by Friday 31st October 2003 to:

Helen Whittaker
Learning and Development
The Chartered Society of Physiotherapy
14 Bedford Row
London WC1R 4ED

or to: whittakerh@csp.org.uk

Thank you very much for your help in producing the CSP whiplash guidelines.

Appendix F:

Analysis of physiotherapists who completed the Delphi questionnaires

Specialist area in physiotherapy	Years spent working in this area	Number of people with WAD seen each year (approx.)	Completed first round yes/no	Completed second round yes/no
Musculoskeletal	7	20	y	n
Out-patients	1	20	y	y
Musculoskeletal (A&E)	2	Not given	y	n
Manager	15	0	y	n
Musculoskeletal (but now manager)	20	None in last 3 years	y	n
Chronic musculoskeletal pain	9	5 (working in HE)	y	y
Out-patients	18	200	y	y
Out-patients (chronic pain/fatigue syndrome)	13 in musculoskeletal of which last 5 in chronic pain	50	y	n
Research	14	50	y	n
Musculoskeletal	15	30	y	n
Spinal disorders	7	10 (much less since closure of casualty dept in hospital)	y	y
Chronic pain	9	not given	y	y
Orthopaedic out-patients	10	100	y	y
Musculoskeletal	20	10	y	y
Musculoskeletal	8	4	y	y
Manipulative diploma graduate	23	50	y	n
Musculoskeletal	10	None at present	y	y
Neuro-musculoskeletal dysfunction	33	Used to be about 1 per week	y	n
Musculoskeletal	16	50–100	y	n
Musculoskeletal	6	30	y	y
Musculoskeletal	4+	10+	y	y
Neuro musculoskeletal	15	15	y	y
Musculoskeletal disorders and rheumatology	9	1–2 (researcher)	y	y
Musculoskeletal	9	10	y	n
Musculoskeletal	10	6–10	y	y

Specialist area in physiotherapy	Years spent working in this area	Number of people with WAD seen each year (approx.)	Completed first round yes/no	Completed second round yes/no
Musculoskeletal	13	5 (currently lecture, in past 50)	y	y
Neck and shoulder in musculoskeletal out-patients	28	40	y	y
Neuro musculoskeletal	9	not given	y	n
Musculoskeletal	6	8	y	y
Musculoskeletal	12	30–40	y	y
Musculoskeletal	15	Less than 10	y	y
Out-patient musculoskeletal	7	150	y	y
Musculoskeletal	15	10–15	y	y
not given	not given	not given	y	y
Exercise prescription/cognitive behavioural approach	3	0	y	y
Musculoskeletal, low back pain	13	20	y	y
Musculoskeletal	15	50	y	y
Orthopaedic/musculoskeletal	10	30–40	y	y
Out-patient/spinal	10	10–15	y	y

Appendix G

The Delphi results are given below as percentages. The numbers responding 'Agree' and 'Strongly agree' have been combined as have the numbers responding 'Disagree' and 'Strongly disagree'.

The raw data from the second Delphi round is available from the Chartered Society of Physiotherapy.

The order of the results in this Appendix is slightly different to the order of the questions in the second Delphi round (Appendix E). The changes have been made to follow the order of the text in the guidelines.

Questions seven and eight in the Delphi questionnaire have been omitted in this Appendix. This is because the GDG disagreed with the Delphi results for these questions, on safety grounds. The questions concerned the circumstances in which tests for instability would be carried out. A fuller response from the GDG can be found in section 3.6.5.7.

Risk factors	Agree %	Neither %	Disagree %	Don't know %
The following indicate increased likelihood of severe symptoms				
Looking to one side during a rear-end collision	85	7	4	4
Poorly positioned headrest	88	4	4	4
These pre-existing factors indicate that a poor prognosis is likely following WAD				
Pre-existing degenerative changes	93	7	0	0
Pre-trauma headaches	59	26	15	0
Pre-trauma neck ache	96	0	4	0
Low level of job satisfaction	85	11	4	0
Injury occurring at 50 years of age and above	48	41	11	0
Being female	26	41	33	0
The following post-injury factors suggest that a poor prognosis is likely following WAD				
Headache for more than six months following injury	96	0	4	0
Neurological signs present after injury	93	0	7	0

The natural history of WAD suggests that				
It is good practice for physiotherapists to advise people with WAD that they are very likely to recover	100	0	0	0

This textbook could be recommend to assist physiotherapists in assessing people with WAD?				
Maitland G, Hengerveld E, Banks K, English K (2001) Maitland's Vertebral Manipulation (6th ed.) Butterworth Heinmann, Oxford.	56	33	7	4

	Agree %	Neither %	Disagree %	Don't know %
Boyling J, Palastanga N (1994) Grieves Modern Manual Therapy 2nd Edition, Churchill Living´stone, Edinburgh.	69	23	4	4
Grieve G P (1988) Common Vertebral Joint Problems Churchill Livingstone, Edinburgh.	56	26	7	11
Petty N J, Moore A P (2001) Neuromusculoskeletal Examination and Assessment: A Handbook for Therapists (2nd ed.) Churchill Livingstone, Edinburgh.	54	23	11	12
Main C, Spanswick CC (2000) Pain Management: an Interdisciplinary Approach Churchill Livingstone, Edinburgh.	67	11	7	15
Oliver J, Middleditch A (1991) Functional Anatomy of the Spine Butterworth Heinmann Oxford.	41	33	15	11
Strong J (2002) Pain a Textbook for Therapists Churchill Livingstone, Edinburgh.	44	19	7	30
Grant R (Ed.) (1994) Physical Therapy of the Cervical and Thoracic Spine (2nd ed.) Churchill Livingstone, New York.	52	18	0	30
Gifford L (ed.) Topical Issues in Pain (series)	85	7	4	4

In the acute stage, entering physiotherapy services is best prioritised by:

	Agree %	Neither %	Disagree %	Don't know %
A physiotherapist working in the accident and emergency department	78	15	7	0
A physiotherapist assessing individual people by telephone	56	33	11	0
A physiotherapist screening individual people using the information provided on the referral form	37	48	15	0
A physiotherapist screening individual people	85	11	4	0

The following factors make an individual person a higher priority at the assessment/screening stage

	Agree %	Neither %	Disagree %	Don't know %
The injury occurred more recently	89	4	7	0
The symptoms have been present over a longer time period	41	33	26	0
Person's activities of daily living are disrupted	96	4	0	0
Person is off work	96	4	0	0

Do these recognised barriers to recovery from chronic pain apply to people with WAD?

	Agree %	Neither %	Disagree %	Don't know %
High fear of pain and movement (fearing that pain and/or movement leads to harm)	100	0	0	0
High tendency to catastrophise (thinking the worst about the pain)	96	4	0	0
Low self-efficacy (lacking confidence in ability to undertake a particular activity)	100	0	0	0
Severe anxiety	100	0	0	0
Evidence of severe depression	100	0	0	0
Low pain locus of control (believing that it is impossible to control the pain)	100	0	0	0
High use of passive coping strategies (withdrawal/passing on responsibility for pain control to others)	100	0	0	0

	Agree %	Neither %	Disagree %	Don't know %
Series of previously failed treatments	92	4	4	0
Person currently off work as a result of the pain	85	11	4	0
Chronic widespread pain	96	0	4	0
Poor understanding of the healing mechanism	80	12	8	0
Non compliance with treatment and advice	88	8	4	0
Problems in relationships with others	92	0	8	0
Negative expectations of treatment	81	15	4	0
Unrealistic expectations of treatment	86	14	0	0
Failure of the physiotherapist to address an individual person's needs	80	20	0	0
Poor clinical reasoning by the physiotherapist	69	31	0	0

The following post-injury factors suggest that a poor prognosis is likely following WAD

	Agree %	Neither %	Disagree %	Don't know %
Unresolved legal issues	81	15	4	0

The barriers to recovery should be assessed at the following stages after injury:

	Agree %	Neither %	Disagree %	Don't know %
Less than 2 weeks after injury	56	18	26	0
After 2 weeks and before 6 weeks	81	8	11	0
After 6 weeks and before 12 weeks	85	11	4	0
At 12 weeks or more	82	7	11	0

A major aim of physiotherapy treatment should be

	Agree %	Neither %	Disagree %	Don't know %
To relieve symptoms	93	7	0	0
To improve function	100	0	0	0
To facilitate empowerment of the person	100	0	0	0
To get the person back to normal activity/work	100	0	0	0

Physiotherapy intervention for WAD in the acute stage
(zero to two weeks after injury)

The following should be used to enhance the effect of rest and analgesia in reducing pain

	Agree %	Neither %	Disagree %	Don't know %
Soft collars	15	11	74	0
Manual mobilisation	48	30	22	0
Active exercise	100	0	0	0
A general active exercise programme	92	4	4	0
An active individual exercise programme following assessment	93	7	0	0
Interferential therapy	7	30	63	0
Ultrasound treatment	11	26	63	0
Massage	33	26	41	0

	Agree %	Neither %	Disagree %	Don't know %
Soft tissue techniques	59	19	22	0
TENS	52	30	18	0
Laser treatment	0	27	65	8
Infrared light	4	11	85	0
Traction	8	16	76	0
Acupuncture	33	33	26	8
Relaxation	52	26	22	0
Education about the origin of the pain	96	4	0	0
Advice about coping strategies	100	0	0	0
The effect of early manual mobilisation techniques versus initial rest and soft collar				
Early manual mobilising is more effective than rest and a soft collar in improving neck range of movement	81	15	4	0
Early manual mobilisation is more effective than initial rest in improving function	81	15	4	0
An early physiotherapy programme versus initial rest and an exercise routine				
Early physiotherapy 'as usual' is more effective than initial rest followed by an exercise routine in improving function.	52	26	18	4

Physiotherapy intervention for WAD in the sub acute stage
(i.e. more than 2 weeks and less than 12 weeks after injury)

Manipulation and manual mobilisation

	Agree %	Neither %	Disagree %	Don't know %
Manipulation alone reduces pain	15	30	55	0
Manual mobilisation alone reduces pain	26	26	48	0
Manual mobilisation is more effective than a combination of ice and TENS in reducing pain	22	45	26	7
Manual mobilisation is more effective than acupuncture in reducing pain	19	45	18	18
Manual mobilisation is more effective than a single manipulation in reducing pain	33	44	19	4
Combined manipulation and manual mobilisation reduces pain	52	40	4	4
Combined manipulation and manual mobilisation is effective in improving function	52	26	18	4
Adverse events resulting from cervical manipulation				
The risk of serious adverse events (e.g. vertebrobasilar accidents) from manipulation is low	93	0	7	0
Minor or moderate adverse events (e.g. headache or nausea) occur in around half of all people receiving cervical manipulation	30	26	33	11

	Agree %	Neither %	Disagree %	Don't know %
The effect of other interventions				
Acupuncture is effective in reducing neck pain	52	19	7	22
Soft collars are effective in reducing pain	19	33	48	0
Education is effective in improving neck function	96	4	0	0
Advice about coping strategies is effective in enabling people to return to normal activities	96	4	0	0
Traction is effective in reducing neck pain	26	22	52	0
TENS is effective in reducing neck pain	59	22	19	0
Infrared light is effective in reducing neck pain	4	29	63	4
Laser treatment is effective in reducing neck pain	4	26	55	15
Interferential therapy is effective in reducing neck pain	11	30	59	0
Ultrasound treatment is effective in reducing neck pain	22	26	52	0
Massage is effective in reducing neck pain	65	23	12	0
Soft tissue techniques are effective in reducing neck pain	78	11	7	4
Muscle retraining and deep neck flexor activity is effective in improving function	78	11	11	0
Phasic exercise (rapid eye-hand-neck movements) is effective in improving function	15	46	12	27

Manipulation and manual mobilisation				
Manual mobilisation reduces pain	78	11	11	0
Manipulation reduces pain	59	30	11	0
Manual mobilisation is as effective as ice in reducing pain	30	48	15	7
Manual mobilisation is more effective than a combination of ice and TENS in reducing pain	33	52	4	11
Manual mobilisation is more effective than acupuncture in reducing pain	11	58	19	12
Manual mobilisation is more effective than a single manipulation in reducing pain	39	46	15	0
Combined manipulation and manual mobilisation reduce pain	70	22	8	0
Combined manipulation and manual mobilisation is effective in improving function	70	15	15	0

Comparing manipulation and exercise combined with manipulation alone				
Manipulation and exercise is more effective than manipulation alone in reducing long term pain	85	11	4	0
Manipulation and exercise is more effective than manipulation alone in terms of patient satisfaction	74	15	4	7

	Agree %	Neither %	Disagree %	Don't know %
Manipulation and exercise is more effective than manipulation alone in improving function	89	4	7	0

Exercise therapy

	Agree %	Neither %	Disagree %	Don't know %
Standard exercise (stretching, isometric, isokinetic) is more effective than phasic exercise (rapid eye-hand-neck movements) in improving function	54	15	0	31
Strengthening exercise is more effective than endurance training in reducing pain	4	66	15	15
Strengthening exercise is more effective than endurance training in improving function	4	60	24	12
Strengthening exercise is more effective than body awareness training in reducing pain	11	54	27	8
Strengthening exercise is more effective than body awareness training in improving function	19	50	19	12
Strengthening exercise is more effective than passive physiotherapy in reducing pain	62	23	11	4
Strengthening exercise is more effective than passive physiotherapy in improving function	76	16	4	4
Group exercise is effective in improving function	68	24	4	4
Proprioceptive exercise improves neck function	73	19	4	4
Neck schools are effective in improving function	39	46	0	15
Extension retraction exercises are effective in improving neck function	58	31	11	0
Mobilising exercises are effective in reducing pain	96	4	0	0
Exercises based on individual patient assessment is more effective than a generalised exercise programme in improving function	92	0	8	0
Advice about coping strategies combined with exercise is more effective than exercise alone in returning to normal activity	100	0	0	0

Acupuncture

	Agree %	Neither %	Disagree %	Don't know %
Acupuncture is more effective than massage in reducing pain	19	48	11	22
Acupuncture is more effective than sham acupuncture in reducing pain	33	19	11	37

Multidisciplinary psychosocial rehabilitation

	Agree %	Neither %	Disagree %	Don't know %
Multidisciplinary rehabilitation is more effective than traditional rehabilitation (physiotherapy, rest, sick leave) in improving function	78	11	0	11

The following outcome measures are likely to be most effective for assessing progress of people with WAD

	Agree %	Neither %	Disagree %	Don't know %
For pain: The visual analogue scale	93	7	0	0
For function: The neck disability index	78	11	0	11
For return to usual activities: The physiotherapy specific functional scale	45	22	0	33
For a patient centred measure: Measure yourself medical outcome profile (MYMOP)	41	15	0	44
For fear of movement: The Tampa Scale for Kinesiophobia (TSK)	12	0	0	88
For quality of life: SF-36	58	15	0	27
For patient satisfaction: The CSPs Clinical Audit tool, The patient feedback questionnaire	26	22	0	52
For anxiety and depression: The hospital anxiety and depression questionnaire	54	15	4	27
For self-efficacy: The Chronic Pain Self-Efficacy Scale (CPSS)	44	15	0	41

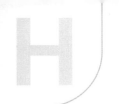

Appendix H

Reproduced by kind permission of Royal College of Radiologists from: RCR Working Party (2003) Making the best use of a department of clinical radiology: guidelines for doctors. 5th ed. Royal College of Radiologists, London.

Indications for x-rays (XR), computed tomography (CT) and magnetic resonance imaging (MRI)

Clinical/diagnostic problem	Investigation	Recommendation	Comment
Conscious person with head and/or facial injuries	XR cervical spine	Indicated only in specific circumstances	XR will not be necessary provided that all five of the following criteria are met: • No midline cervical tenderness • No focal neurological deficit • Normal alertness • No intoxication • No painful distracting injury.
Unconscious person with head injury	XR cervical spine, CT	Indicated	Good quality XRs should demonstrate the whole of the cervical spine down to T1/2. If the cervico-thoracic junction is not clearly seen or there are any possible areas of fracture then CT is required. Where available, spiral CT may be used as an alternative to XR, and is essential if the cervico-thoracic junction is not clearly seen on XR. Both techniques may be difficult in the severely traumatised person, and manipulation must be avoided.
Neck Injury with pain	XR cervical spine	Indicated	Discuss with department of clinical radiology.
	CT / MRI	Specialised investigation	May be valuable when XR is equivocal or lesion complex.
Neck injury with neurological deficit	XR cervical spine	Indicated	For orthopaedic assessment. XR must be of good quality to allow accurate interpretation.
	MRI	Indicated	MRI is the best and safest method of demonstrating intrinsic cord damage, cord compression, ligamentous injuries, and vertebral fractures at multiple levels.
	CT	Specialised investigation	CT myelography may be considered if MRI is not practicable.
Neck injury with pain but XR initially normal; suspected ligamentous injury	XR cervical spine	Specialised investigation	Views taken in flexion and extension (consider fluoroscopy) as achieved by the person with no assistance and under medical supervision.
	MRI	Specialised Investigation	MRI demonstrates ligamentous injuries.

Clinical/diagnostic problem	Investigation	Recommendation	Comment
Possible atlanto-axial subluxation	XR	Indicated	A single lateral cervical spine XR with the person in supervised comfortable flexion should reveal any significant subluxation in person with rheumatoid arthritis, Downs syndrome etc.
	MRI	Specialised investigation	MRI in flexion/extension shows effect on cord when XR is positive or neurological signs are present.
Neck pain, brachialgia, degenerative change	XR	Indicated only in specific circumstances	Neck pain generally improves or resolves with conservative treatment. Degenerative changes begin in early middle age and are often unrelated to symptoms.
	MRI	Specialised investigation	Consider MRI and specialist referral when pain affects lifestyle or when there are neurological signs. CT myelography may occasionally be required to provide further delineation or when MRI is unavailable or impossible.

Indicated is an investigation most likely to contribute to clinical diagnosis and management.

Specialised investigation – frequently complex, time-consuming or resource-intensive investigation which will usually only be performed after discussion with the radiologist or in the context of locally agreed protocols.

Indicated only in specific circumstances – non routine studies which will only be carried out if a clinician provides cogent reasons or if the radiologist feels the examination represents an appropriate way of furthering the diagnosis and management of the patient.

Appendix I

Clinical guidelines for the physiotherapy management of whiplash associated disorder (WAD)

Reviewers' comments

We will acknowledge all reviewers in the guidelines. Please include details that you would like including in the final publication in the table below.

Name	Qualifications	Post	Speciality
	MCSP etc.	e.g. senior II physiotherapist	e.g. muscuolskeletal physiotherapy

Please aim to make a general comment on each of the following.

Are the guidelines readable?

Are there any major concerns or issues that you would like to raise?

Do you think that the guidelines are clinically relevant?

What are the implications for your trust / university / other employer (please indicate which you are referring to)

What comments can you make on the presentation of the guidelines?

Are there omissions?

Please note specific points, inaccuracies or typing errors in the table below:

Page	comment

Please continue on another sheet of paper if you have further comments

Appendix J

Reflective practice record for WAD

1. Describe a practice-based event

2. How did you respond to the event (thoughts, actions feelings)?

3. Why did you respond as you did?

What specific issues does the event raise in relation to question/s posed in the WAD guidelines?

4. Relevant WAD question/s (Section 4)

5. Evidence-based practice issues:

6. Clinical relevance issues:

7. WAD recommendation issues:

From this event, what have you learnt about:

8. Formal decision-making?

9. Intuitive decision-making?

10. Ethical decision-making?

Appendix K

Glossary and abbreviations

Term	Meaning
Accessory movements	Joint movements that cannot be performed voluntarily or in isolation by the patient.
Acupuncture	Procedure of Chinese origin involving the insertion of thin needles into certain areas of the body to relieve pain.
Acute (stage of WAD)	Symptoms in the first two weeks after injury.
Adson manoeuvre	A test for thoracic outlet syndrome. Also known as Adson's Test.
Aetiology	The causes of a disease or abnormal condition.
Allen's test	A test for occlusion of the radial or ulnar artery.
Analgesic ladder	The order in which analgesic drugs should be tried e.g. (1) Non-opioid drugs e.g. aspirin, paracetamol, NSAIDs (2) Weak opioids e.g. Codeine (3) Strong opioids e.g. morphine, diamorphine.
Behavioural therapy	A psychological treatment that aims to remove conditioned responses to symptoms, whatever the underlying diagnosis. Desensitisation, operant conditioning, and aversion therapy are examples of behavioural therapy.
Biomedical	Relating to the biological and medical sciences.
Blinding	Concealment of treatments in a randomised controlled trial from trial participants, clinicians and/or outcome assessors to reduce biases for or against particular treatments, that may influence the outcomes.
Black flags	The actual barriers preventing a person from returning to work.
Blue flags	A person's perception of the barriers preventing them from returning to work.
Brachialgia	Severe pain in the arm.
Catastrophising	A person viewing their situation with a catastrophic outcome, e.g. someone thinking that the neck pain they have had for a few weeks will lead to a chronic condition.
Chartered Society of Physiotherapy (CSP)	The professional body for physiotherapists in the UK.
Chiropractic treatment	Based on the theory that a person's state of health is determined by the condition of the nervous system. The most important component is the manual treatment of joints and muscles.
Chronic (stage of WAD)	Persistent symptoms lasting more than 12 weeks after injury.
Clonus	A rapid succession of relaxations and contractions of a muscle usually resulting from a sustained stretching stimulus.
Cochrane Collaboration	An international non-profit and independent organisation producing and disseminating systematic reviews of healthcare interventions. The Cochrane Database of Systematic Reviews and other useful databases are published on The Cochrane Library.
Cognition	The mental process of knowing, including thinking, reasoning, learning and judging.

Cognitive behavioural therapy	A talking therapy conducted by a trained therapist that identifies and modifies negative patterns of thinking, changes emotional responses and behaviour.
Controlled clinical trial	A prospective, experimental study that compares a group of people that are given a therapy of interest with at least one other control group, who are usually given standard therapy, a placebo/sham therapy or no treatment.
Coping strategies	A person's style, or strategy for coping with situations that involve psychological stress or threat.
Correlation study	A statistical study that examines the degree in which one random variable is associated with or can be predicted from another.
CT (Computed Tomography) scan	A special radiographic technique that uses a computer to assimilate multiple X-ray images into a 2 dimensional cross-sectional image.
Delphi method	An iterative method of gaining consensus agreement from experts or other individuals on a topic for which there is inconsistent, little or no empirical evidence.
Double blind	Same as Blinding, however both trial participants and clinicians are unaware of the therapy received.
Dynamic resisted exercises	Exercise where movement is resisted through a range.
Dysarthria	Weakness or lack of coordination of the muscles required for speech, preventing clear pronunciation of words.
Dysphagia	Difficulty swallowing.
Electroacupuncture	A form of acupuncture using low frequency electrically stimulated needles to produce analgesia and anaesthesia and to treat disease.
Electrotherapy	The therapeutic use of electrophysical agents.
EMG (Electromyography) biofeedback	Recording of a muscle's electrical activity.
Epidemiology	The study of the causes, prevalence and spread of disease in a community.
Extension retraction exercises	Active exercises for the upper cervical atlanto-occipital region (chin tucks).
External validity	The extent to which a research finding is generalisable to the population at large.
Fear avoidance	Avoidance of activity resulting from a person's belief that the experience of pain will lead to further damage and or (re)injury.
Fibromyalgia	A disorder characterised by musculoskeletal pain, spasms, stiffness, fatigue and severe sleep disturbances.
Guideline development group (GDG)	Team of clinical experts, research methodologists, patient representatives and administrators who work to produce a guideline.
Health Professions Council (HPC)	An independent, UK-wide, regulatory body that is responsible for setting and maintaining standards of professional training, performance and conduct for healthcare professions, including the physiotherapy.
Hydrotherapy	Physiotherapy treatment performed in water, utilising its physical properties.
Hypothesis	An assumption made in advance, which is formally tested using statistical tests to confirm, modify or disprove it.

Ice therapy	Treating injuries with ice.
Infrared light therapy	Treatment using different types of infrared radiation, such as heating pads or incandescent lights.
Instability tests	Specific tests to check the structural integrity of the upper cervical ligament complex.
Intention-to-treat	Participants in a clinical trial are analysed according to the treatment the randomisation process allocated them to, whether they received that treatment or not.
Interferential therapy	A medium frequency electrical modality transmitted using surface electrodes designed to increase circulation and decrease pain.
Interscapular	The section of the upper back between the shoulders.
In vivo	In a living body. Usually refers to studies conducted within a living organism.
In vitro	Outside the living body and in an artificial or laboratory environment e.g. in a test tube.
Isokinetic exercise	Exercise performed with an apparatus that provides variable resistance to a movement, in order to maintain a constant speed no matter how much effort is exerted. Such exercise is used to test and improve muscular strength and endurance.
Isometric exercise	Exercises that contract the muscles without moving the involved parts of the body in order to improve fitness and build up muscle strength.
Kinaesthetic sensibility	Awareness of movement within the body. See also Proprioception.
Kinesophobia	A debilitating fear of movement resulting from a feeling of vulnerability to a painful injury or reinjury.
Laser	A medical instrument that produces a powerful beam of light, which can emit intense heat when focused at close range.
Likert scale	A point scoring system often used to measure attitudes by asking respondents the degree with which they agree with statements. For example, strongly agree, no opinion or strongly disagree.
Locus of control	The extent to which a person feels in control of things around them and their own behaviour.
Lordosis	Forward curvature of the spine normally occurring in the cervical and lumbar regions.
Lhermittes sign	Sudden electric-like shocks radiating down the arms, trunk or legs on head and neck flexion, which is sometimes seen in cervical cord compression.
Maitland principles	A concept of manipulative physiotherapy.
Manipulative therapy	The passive, sometimes forceful movement of bones, joints and soft tissues carried out by trained therapists, usually to relieve pain, reduce joint stiffness or correct deformity. Manipulation and manual mobilisation are forms of manipulative therapy.
Manipulation	A high velocity, small amplitude thrust performed by the therapist at the end of the available range of movement that is not under the control of the patient.

Manual mobilisation	Small rhythmical oscillations or sustained pressure by the therapist within the range of movement that can be resisted by the patient if the procedure becomes too painful.
Massage	Systematic rubbing of the skin and deeper tissues. Massage helps to improve circulation, prevent scarring in injured tissues, relax muscle spasms, improve muscle tone and reduce swelling.
McKenzie method	A concept of assessment and treatment of the spine. A musculoskeletal approach to management.
Mechanical neck disorders	Non-specific neck problems with an absence of red flags and known pathology.
Motor control	The ability of the central nervous system to direct and control movement.
MRI (Magnetic Resonance Imaging)	Magnetic fields and radio frequencies are used to produce clear images of body tissue.
Multidisciplinary	Involving professionals from several disciplines, such as physiotherapists, orthopaedic surgeons, nurses, psychologists, etc.
Multimodal treatment	A treatment programme including different modalities e.g. exercise, manual mobilisation and education.
Myelography	An invasive procedure that involves injecting a radio-opaque substance into the spinal cord in order to assist in the diagnosis of diseases of the spine or spinal cord.
National Health Service (NHS)	The government-led health system in the UK.
National Institute for Health and Clinical Excellence	An independent organisation funded by the NHS responsible for providing national guidance on the promotion of good health and the prevention and treatment of ill health.
Neck schools	A concept of group treatment programmes to treat neck pain.
Neurological	Relating to the nervous system.
Nociception	The sensation of feeling pain.
Non steroidal anti-inflammatory drugs (NSAIDs)	A large group of drugs, including aspirin and ibuprofen, that relieve pain and reduce inflammation by prohibiting the formation of prostaglandins.
Nystagmus	Involuntary, rapid, rhythmic eye movements.
Outcome	The result of treatment of a patient or client.
Outcome measure	A validated test or scale for measuring a particular outcome of interest in order to assess the effectiveness of a therapy or service.
Outcome assessment	The process of measuring an outcome using an outcome measure.
Paraesthesia	Experiencing an unusual sensation, e.g. tingling, burning, itching, etc.
Passive accessory intervertebral movement (PAIVM)	Investigation of accessory gliding movements (joint movements that cannot be performed voluntarily or in isolation) in a joint.

Passive movement	Any movement of a joint which is produced by any means other than the particular muscles related to that particular joint movement. It includes both mobilization and manipulation.
Passive physiological intervertebral movement (PPIVM)	Investigation of passive physiological movements (joint movements that could be performed voluntarily or in isolation) to confirm restrictions seen on active movement testing.
Patient empowerment	Enabling patients to participate in decisions about health care. This can be either on a personal level, making decisions about their own care or as a member of the public in the planning, provision and monitoring of health care services.
PEDro (Physiotherapy Evidence Database)	Database of randomised controlled clinical trials, systematic reviews and evidence-based clinical practice guidelines in physiotherapy.
Phasic exercises	Exercise involving rapid eye-hand-neck-arm movements.
Physical agents	A physiotherapy modality that is not manual e.g. electrotherapy and ice.
Physical therapy	The use of physical approaches to promote, maintain and restore physical, psychological and social well-being. Alternative term for physiotherapy.
Placebo	An inactive treatment made to look and feel the same as an active treatment. It is usually given to the control group in a randomised controlled trial in order to mask which treatment the patient has received and therefore reduce any potential bias.
PRODIGY guidance	Source of clinical knowledge based on the best available evidence about common conditions and symptoms managed in primary care.
Prognostic factors	Factors that can be used to predict the patient's outcome or the course their recovery will take.
Proprioception	The reception of stimuli from within the body, including sense of position (e.g. the awareness of the joints at rest) and kinaesthesia (see Kinaesthetic).
Psychopathology	The study of the causes, processes and manifestations of mental disorders.
Psychosocial	Combination of psychological and social factors.
Pulsed electromagnetic therapy (PEMT)	A generic term for treatment using pulsed-electromagnetic energy.
p-value (p=)	The level of statistical significance of the results in a statistical test. It is the probability that the results observed could have occurred by chance. A p-value of less than 0.05 is generally considered as statistically significant. See Statistically significant.
Quasi-	Almost, seemingly.
Quasi-randomised	Randomising trial participants to groups using a method that is not completely random, e.g. even and odd hospital numbers or alternate patients. See Randomised controlled trial.
Randomised controlled trial (RCT)	A clinical trial comparing two or more groups of people, who are given different treatments or interventions. People are allocated to groups at random (see Randomisation) and, if possible, the trial subjects and those measuring the outcomes are not aware which treatment is allocated to which subject (see Blinding).

Randomisation	Assigning participants in a randomised controlled trial to treatment groups on a random basis in an attempt to ensure the groups are balanced.
Red flags	Factors that may indicate serious pathology.
Reflective practice	Professional activity in which the practitioner thinks critically about practice and as a result may modify practice or behaviour and/or modify learning needs.
Rehabilitation	Helping individuals regain skills and abillities that have been lost as a result of illness, injury or disease in order to maximise their physical, mental and social functioning.
Relaxation exercises	Exercises to address muscle tension that accompanies pain.
Reliability	The extent to which the results of a study can be reproduced if the study is carried out again exactly as reported.
Self efficacy	An individual's belief that he or she is capable of successfully performing a certain set of behaviours.
Shaken baby syndrome	Severe whiplash-type injuries observed in babies or children who have been shaken violently, causing retinal haemorrhages or convulsions, which could lead to intercranial bleeding from tearing of cerebral blood vessels.
Sham	A dummy procedure made to look and feel like an active therapy. See Placebo.
Short-wave diathermy	High frequency, short-wave electrical currents with a wavelength of 11.062 metres, used to provide heat deep into the body.
Single blinded	When either the patient or the person measuring clinical outcomes in a clinical trial is unaware of the treatment being given to the patient. See Blinding.
Slump test	A test that combines cervical/trunk flexion, straight leg raise (SLR) and ankle dorsiflexion and is used to assess neural tension by reproducing the subject's symptoms.
Soft collar	Foam neck brace used to restrict movement of the head and neck.
Soft tissue techniques	Usually manual techniques used to treat soft tissues and related neural and vascular components in the body.
Somatisation	Process by which psychological events or needs are expressed as physical symptoms.
Statistically significant	The results of a study have probably not occurred by chance and a true difference has been observed.
Subacute (stage of WAD)	Symptoms lasting more than two weeks and up to 12 weeks since injury.
Supine	Lying on the back, face upwards.
Systematic review	A scientific method for identifying, appraising, synthesising and communicating all the available research on a particular topic using pre-determined criteria.
Transcutaneous Electrical Nerve Stimulation (TENS)	The use of electrical fields via electrodes applied through the skin in order to relieve pain.
Thermotherapy	Using heat or cold as a treatment for disease or injury.
Thoracic outlet syndrome	Pain, numbness, tingling, and/or weakness in the arm and hand due to pressure on the nerves or blood vessels supplying the arm. Muscles and ligaments become tight or bony abnormalities form in the thoracic outlet area of the body i.e. behind the collar bone.

Traction	A manual or mechanical modality to distract joint surfaces. It can either be intermittent or a sustained force.
Trigger point	A highly sensitive point within the muscle or myofascial tissue, that produces a painful response when stimulated with touch, pain or pressure.
Ultrasound	The diagnostic or therapeutic use of high-frequency sound waves to produce a mechanical effect and/or heat.
Upper limb tension test (ULTT)	Test used to assess the neural mobility of the upper quadrant.
Validity	The extent to which a research finding is accurate and measures what it purports to measure.
Vertebrobasilar	Refers to the vertebral and basilar arteries at the base of the brain.
Visual analogue scale (VAS)	A scale used to provide a quantitative measure of a subjective outcome, such as pain. The scale is usually a 10cm line with definitions at either end, e.g. no pain at 0cm and worse pain ever felt at the 10cm end. The patient is asked to indicate where, on the line, best describes their pain.
Whiplash associated disorder (WAD)	A variety of symptoms that result from bony and/or soft tissue injuries sustained in a whiplash injury.
Yellow flags	Psychological and sociological factors that may predict chronicity i.e. long-term disability and work-loss.
Zygapophyseal joints	Synovial joints between articular processes of the vertebrae. Also known as facet joints.

Bibliography

The following resources were used in compiling this glossary:

Bottomley, JM (ed) (2002). *Quick reference dictionary for physical therapy (2nd edition).* Slack Incorporated, New Jersey

Churchill's illustrated medical dictionary (1989). Churchill Livingstone, New York

Hutchinson, DR (2002). *Dictionary of clinical research (3rd edition).* Brookwood Medical Publications Ltd, Richmond

Hyperdictionary. Available from: http://www.hyperdictionary.com/ (accessed 9th June 2005)

Mosby's medical, nursing, & allied health dictionary (6th edition) (2001) Mosby, St Louis

National Electronic Library for Health. Dictionaries and Internet searching. Available from: http://www.nelh.nhs.uk/directories.asp (accessed 9th June 2005)

Khan, KS, ter Riet, G, Glanville, J, Sowden, A, Kleijnen, J (editors) (2001). *Undertaking systematic reviews of research on effectiveness.* CRD Report 4, (2nd edition) NHS Centre for Reviews and Dissemination, 2001, York

Porter, S (ed) (2005). *Dictionary of physiotherapy.* Elsevier Butterworth Heinemann. London

University of Newcastle upon Tyne. On-line medical dictionary. Available from: http://cancerweb.ncl.ac.uk/cgi-bin/omd?action=Home&query= (accessed 9th June 2005)

Appendix L

References in Alphabetical Order

The references in section 14 of this guideline are given below in alphabetical order by first author.

The numbering refers to the reference number in the text, section 14 and appendix B.

214　Agencie Nationale d'Acreditation et d'Evaluation en Sante (2003). *Physiotherapy in common neck pain and whiplash*. Available from: http://www.anaes.fr/anaes/anaesparametrage.nsf/Page?ReadForm&Section=/anaes/SiteWeb.nsf/wRubriquesID/APEH-3YTFUH?OpenDocument&Defaut=y& (Assessed on 6th May 2005)

56　AGREE Collaboration (2001). *AGREE Instrument: Appraisal of guidelines for research and evaluation*. The AGREE Collaboration. Available from: http://www.agreecollaboration.org (Assessed on 6th May 2005)

150　Albright, J, Allman, R, Bonfiglio, RP, Conill, A, Dobkin, B, Guccione, AA, Hasson, SM, Russo, R, Shekelle, P, Susman, JL, Brosseau, L, Tugwell, P, Wells, GA, Robinson, VA, Graham, ID, Shea, BJ, McGowan, J, Peterson, J, Poulin, L, Tousignant, M, Corriveau, H, Morin, M, Pelland, L, Laferriere, L, Casimiro, L and Tremblay, LE (2001). Philadelphia panel evidence-based clinical practice guidelines on selected rehabilitation interventions for neck pain. *Physical Therapy* **81** (10), 1701–1717

50　Alder, M and Ziglio, E (1996). *Gazing into the oracle. The Delphi method and its application to social policy and public health*. Jessica Kingsley, London.

116　Amundson, GM (1994). The evaluation and treatment of cervical whiplash. *Current Opinion in Orthopedics* **5** (2), 17–27

193　Anderson, KO, Dowds, BN, Pelletz, RE, Edwards, WT and Peeters-Asdourian, C (1995). Development and initial validation of a scale to measure self-efficacy beliefs in patients with chronic pain. *Pain* **63** (1), 77–84

190　Aylard, PR, Gooding, JH, McKenna, PJ and Snaith, RP (1987). A validation study of three anxiety and depression self-assessment scales. *Journal of Psychosomatic Research* **31** (2), 261–268

164　Baker, SM, Marshak, HH, Rice, GT and Zimmerman, GJ (2001). Patient participation in physical therapy goal setting. *Physical Therapy* **81** (5), 1118–1126

172　Bandura, A and Walter, RH (1963). *Social learning and personality development*. Thinehart & Winston, New York

114　Banic, B, Petersen-Felix, S, Andersen, OK, Radanov, BP, Villiger, PM, Arendt Nielsen, L and Curatolo, M (2004). Evidence for spinal cord hypersensitivity in chronic pain after whiplash injury and in fibromyalgia. *Pain* **107** (1–2), 7–15

82　Barancik, JI, Kramer, CF and Thode, HC (1989). *Epidemiology of motor vehicle injuries in Suffolk County, New York before and after enactment of the New York State seat belt use law*. US Department of Transportation, National Highway Traffic Safety Administration, Washington DC

134　Barker, S, Kesson, M, Ashmore, J, Turner, G, Conway, J and Stevens, D (2000). Guidance for pre-manipulative testing of the cervical spine. *Manual Therapy* **5** (1), 37–40

119　Barnsley, L, Lord, S and Bogduk, N (1994). Whiplash injury. *Pain* **58** (3), 283–307

159　Barr, J and Threlkeld, AJ (2000). Patient – practitioner collaboration in clinical decision-making. *Physiotherapy Research International* **5** (4), 254–260

215　Bekkering, G, Hendriks HJM , Lanser K, Oostendorp RAB, Scholten-Peeters GGM, Verhagen A P and van der Windt DAWM (2003). Clinical practice guidelines for physical therapy in patients with whiplash-associated disorders. In *Clinical Practice Guidelines in the Netherlands: a prospect for continuous quality improvement in Physical Therapy*. Royal Dutch Society for Physical Therapy, Amersfoort

195   Bekkering, GE (2004). *Physiotherapy guidelines for low back pain: development, implementation and evaluation, (PhD thesis).* Dutch Institute of Allied Health Care and the Institute for Research in Extramural Medicine (EMGO Institute) of the VU University Medical Centre

211   Bekkering, GE, Engers, AJ, Wensing, M, Hendriks, HJ, van Tulder, M, Oostendorp, RA and Bouter, LM (2003). Development of an implementation strategy for physiotherapy guidelines on low back pain. *Australian Journal of Physiotherapy* **49** (3), 208–214

209   Bero, L, Grilli, R, Grimshaw, J and Oxman, AD (1998). *The Cochrane effective practice and organisation of care review group.* In Cochrane Library, Update Software, Oxford.

14   Binder, A (2002). Neck pain. *Clinical Evidence* (7), 1049–1062

118   Bodguk, N (1986). The anatomy and pathophysiology of whiplash. *Clinical Biomechanics* **1** (2), 92–101

69   Bogduk, N (1999). The neck. *Baillieres Best Practice and Research in Clinical Rheumatology* **13** (2), 261–285

16   Bogduk, N (2002). Manual therapy produces greater relief of neck pain than physiotherapy or general practitioner care. *Australian Journal of Physiotherapy* **48**, 240

111   Bogduk, N and Lord, S (1998). Cervical spine disorders. *Current Opinion in Rheumatology* **10** (2), 110–115

61   Bogduk, N and Yoganandan, N (2001). Biomechanics of the cervical spine Part 3: minor injuries. *Clinical Biomechanics* **16** (4), 267–275

32   Bonk, AD, Ferrari, R, Giebel, GD, Edelmann, M and Huser, R (2000). Prospective, randomized, controlled study of activity versus collar, and the natural history for whiplash injury, in Germany. World Congress on whiplash-associated disorders, Vancouver, British Columbia, Canada. February 1999. *Journal of Musculoskeletal Pain* **8** (1–2), 123–132

33   Borchgrevink, G, Kaasa, A, McDonagh, D, Stiles, TC, Haraldseth, O and Lereim, I (1998). Acute treatment of whiplash neck sprain injuries: a randomized trial of treatment during the first 14 days after a car accident. *Spine* **23** (1), 25–31

137   Borchgrevink, G, Smevik, O, Haave, I, Haraldseth, O, Nordby, A and Lereim, I (1997). MRI of cerebrum and cervical columna within two days after whiplash neck sprain injury. *Injury* **28** (5–6), 331–335

84   Bourbeau, R, Desjardins, D, Maag, U and Laberge-Nadeau, C (1993). Neck injuries among belted and unbelted occupants of the front seat of cars. *Journal of Trauma* **35** (5), 794–799

54   Boyce, W, Gowland, C, Russell, D, Goldsmith, C, Rosenbaum, P, Plews, N and Lane, M (1993). Consensus methodology in the development and content validation of a gross motor performance measure. *Physiotherapy Canada* **45** (2), 94–100

127   Boyling, JD and Palastanga, N (1998). *Grieve's modern manual therapy.* Churchill Livingstone, London

55   Bramwell, L and Hykawy, E (1999). The Delphi Technique: a possible tool for predicting future events in nursing education. *Canadian Journal of Nursing Research* **30** (4), 47–58

93   Bring, G, Bjornstig, U and Westman, G (1996). Gender patterns in minor head and neck injuries: an analysis of casualty register data. *Accident Analysis and Prevention* **28** (3), 359–369

109   Brison, RJ, Hartling, L and Pickett, W (2000). A prospective study of acceleration-extension injuries following rear-end motor vehicle collisions. World Congress on whiplash-associated disorders in Vancouver, British Columbia, Canada. February 1999. *Journal of Musculoskeletal Pain* **8** (1–2), 97–113

163   Brody, DS, Miller, SM, Lerman, CE, Smith, DG and Caputo, GC (1989). Patient perception of involvement in medical care: relationship to illness attitudes and outcomes. *Journal of General Internal Medicine* **4** (6), 506–511

151   Bronfort, G, Evans, R, Nelson, B, Aker, PD, Goldsmith, C and Vernon, H (2001). A randomized clinical trial of exercise and spinal manipulation for patients with chronic neck pain. *Spine* **26** (7), 788–797

3   Burton, K (2003). *Treatment guidelines: Is there a need?* In: Proceedings of Whiplash conference 2003, Bath, England. 6–8 May 2003. Lyons Davidson Solicitors, 2003, Bristol

65   Centeno, C (2003). *Whiplash prognosis.* In: Proceedings of Whiplash conference 2003, Bath, England. 6–8 May 2003. Lyons Davidson Solicitors, 2003, Bristol

45   Centre for Evidence-Based Physiotherapy (1999). *The PEDro scale.* Centre for Evidence-Based Physiotherapy, Sydney. Available from: http://www.pedro.fhs.usyd.edu.au/scale_item.html (Accessed 2nd June 2005)

94   Chapline, JF, Ferguson, SA, Lillis, RP, Lund, AK and Williams, AF (2000). Neck pain and head restraint position relative to the driver's head in rear-end collisions. *Accident Analysis and Prevention* **32** (2), 287–297

187   Chartered Society of Physiotherapy (2000). *Clinical audit tools.* The Chartered Society of Physiotherapy, London

194   Chartered Society of Physiotherapy (2000). *Reports for legal purposes: Information paper number PA1.* The Chartered Society of Physiotherapy, London

157   Chartered Society of Physiotherapy (2002). *Rules of professional conduct.* Chartered Society of Physiotherapy, London

48   Chartered Society of Physiotherapy (2003). *Guidance for developing clinical guidelines.* The Chartered Society of Physiotherapy, London. Available from: http://www.csp.org.uk/libraryandinformation/publications/view.cfm?id=275 (Accessed 6th May 2005)

123   Chartered Society of Physiotherapy (2005). *Core standards.* The Chartered Society of Physiotherapy, London

125   Clinical Standards Advisory Group (CSAG) (1994). *Back pain.* HMSO, London

106   Cote, P, Cassidy, JD, Carroll, L, Frank, JW and Bombardier, C (2001). A systematic review of the prognosis of acute whiplash and a new conceptual framework to synthesize the literature. *Spine* **26** (19), E445–458

5   Cote, P, Hogg-Johnson, S, Cassidy, JD, Carroll, L and Frank, JW (2001). The association between neck pain intensity, physical functioning, depressive symptomatology and time-to-claim-closure after whiplash. *Journal of Clinical Epidemiology* **54** (3), 275–286

87   Croft, PR, Lewis, M, Papageorgiou, AC, Thomas, E, Jayson, MI, Macfarlane, GJ and Silman, AJ (2001). Risk factors for neck pain: a longitudinal study in the general population. *Pain* **93** (3), 317–325

183   Crombez, G, Vlaeyen, JW, Heuts, PH and Lysens, R (1999). Pain-related fear is more disabling than pain itself: evidence on the role of pain-related fear in chronic back pain disability. *Pain* **80** (1–2), 329–339

57   Crowe, H (1928). *Injuries to the cervical spine.* In Annual meeting of Western Orthopaedic Association, San Francisco, California

115   Curatolo, M, Petersen-Felix, S, Arendt-Nielsen, L, Giani, C, Zbinden, AM and Radanov, BP (2001). Central hypersensitivity in chronic pain after whiplash injury. *Clinical Journal of Pain* **17** (4), 306–315

142   Dabbs, V and Lauretti, WJ (1995). A risk assessment of cervical manipulation vs. NSAIDs for the treatment of neck pain. *Journal of Manipulative and Physiological Therapeutics* **18** (8), 530–536

130   Dall'Alba, PT, Sterling, MM, Treleaven, JM, Edwards, SL and Jull, G (2001). Cervical range of motion discriminates between asymptomatic persons and those with whiplash. *Spine* **26** (19), 2090–2094

156   Department of Health (2000). *The NHS plan.* Department of Health, London

122   Department of Health (2001). *Department of Health Guide: Reference guide to consent for examination or treatment.* Department of Health, London. Available from: www.dh.gov.uk/PublicationsAndStatistics/Publications/PublicationsPolicyAndGuidance/Publication sPolicyAndGuidanceArticle/fs/en?CONTENT_ID=4006757&chk=snmdw8 (Accessed 6th May 2005)

80   Dolinis, J (1997). Risk factors for 'whiplash' in drivers: a cohort study of rear-end traffic crashes. *Injury* **28** (3), 173–179

201   Doughty, GM and Foster, NE (2003). *Overcoming dissemination and implementation barriers to using clinical practice guidelines in physiotherapy.* Poster presentation in Defining Practice: The Chartered Society of Physiotherapy annual congress. 16–19 October. Birmingham, London

206   Eccles, M, McColl, E, Steen, N, Rousseau, N, Grimshaw, J, Parkin, D and Purves, I (2002). Effect of computerised evidence based guidelines on management of asthma and angina in adults in primary care: cluster randomised controlled trial. *British Medical Journal* **325** (7370), 941

58   Eck, JC, Hodges, SD and Humphreys, SC (2001). Whiplash: a review of a commonly misunderstood injury. *American Journal of Medicine* **110** (8), 651–656

207   Evans, DW, Foster, NE, Vogel, S and Breen, AC (2003). *Implementing evidence-based practice in the UK physical therapy professions: Do they want it and do they need it?* Poster presentation at 6th International forum for low back pain research in primary care, Linkping, Sweden. May 2003

27   Evans, R, Bronfort, G, Nelson, B and Goldsmith, C (2002). Two-year follow-up of a randomized clinical trial of spinal manipulation and two types of exercise for patients with chronic neck pain. *Spine* **27**, 2383–2389

161   Ewles, L and Simnett, I (1992). *Promoting health a practical guide.* Scutari Press, London

198   Feder, G (1994). Management of mild hypertension: which guidelines to follow? *British Medical Journal* **308**, 470–471

197   Feder, G, Eccles, M, Grol, R, Griffiths, C and Grimshaw, J (1999). Clinical guidelines: using clinical guidelines. *British Medical Journal* **318** (7185), 728–730

9   Ferrari, R and Russell, AS (1999). Epidemiology of whiplash: an international dilemma. *Annals of the Rheumatic Diseases* **58** (1), 1–5

10   Field, MJ and Lohr, KNE (1992). *Guidelines for clinical practice: from development to use.* National Academy Press, Washington DC

34   Fitz-Ritson, D (1995). Phasic exercises for cervical rehabilitation after "whiplash" trauma. *Journal of Manipulative and Physiological Therapeutics* **18** (1), 21–24

35   Foley-Nolan, D, Moore, K, Codd, M, Barry, C, O'Connor, P and Coughlan, RJ (1992). Low energy high frequency pulsed electromagnetic therapy for acute whiplash injuries. A double blind randomized controlled study. *Scandinavian Journal of Rehabilitation Medicine* **24** (1), 51–59

200   Foster, NE and Doughty, GM (2003). *Dissemination and implementation of back pain guidelines: perspectives of musculoskeletal physiotherapists and managers.* Paper presented at *6th* International forum for low back pain research in primary care. Linkping, Sweden. May 2003

208   Freemantle, N, Harvey, E, Grimshaw, J, Wolf, F, Bero, L and Grilli, R (1996). *The effectiveness of printed educational materials in changing the behaviour of health care professionals.* In Cochrane Library, Update Software, Oxford

68   Galasko, CS, Murray, PA and Pitcher, M (2000). Prevalence and long-term disability following whiplash-associated disorder. World Congress on whiplash-associated disorders, Vancouver, British Columbia, Canada. February 1999. *Journal of Musculoskeletal Pain* **8** (1–2), 15–27

7   Galasko, CS, Murray, PM, Pitcher, M, Chambers, H, Mansfield, S, Madden, M, Jordon, C, Kinsella, A and Hodson, M (1993). Neck sprains after road traffic accidents: a modern epidemic. *Injury* **24** (3), 155–157

36   Gennis, P, Miller, L, Gallagher, EJ, Giglio, J, Carter, W and Nathanson, N (1996). The effect of soft cervical collars on persistent neck pain in patients with whiplash injury. *Academic Emergency Medicine* **3** (6), 568–573

138   Gotzsche, PC (2002). Non-steroidal anti-inflammatory drugs. *Clinical Evidence* (7), 1063–1070

191   Greenough, CG and Fraser, RD (1991). Comparison of eight psychometric instruments in unselected patients with back pain. *Spine* **16** (9), 1068–1074

199   Grimshaw, J (2001). Changing provider behaviour: an overview of systematic reviews of interventions. *Medical Care* **39** (8)

212   Grol, R and Jones, R (2000). Twenty years of implementation research. *Family Practice* **17** Suppl 1, 32–35

140   Gross, AR, Kay, TM, Kennedy, C, Gasner, D, Hurley, L, Yardley, K, Hendry, L and McLaughlin, L (2002a). Clinical practice guideline on the use of manipulation or mobilization in the treatment of adults with mechanical neck disorders. *Manual Therapy* **7** (4), 193–205

147   Gross, AR, Aker, PD, Goldsmith, C and Peloso, P (2002b). *Patient education for mechanical neck disorders.* The Cochrane Library: Update Software, Oxford

149   Gross, AR, Aker, PD, Goldsmith, C and Peloso, P (2002c). *Physical medicine modalities for mechanical neck disorders.* The Cochrane Library: Update Software, Oxford

100   Grossi, G, Soares, JJ, Angesleva, J and Perski, A (1999). Psychosocial correlates of long-term sick-leave among patients with musculoskeletal pain. *Pain* **80** (3), 607–619

196   Haines, A and Donald, A (1998). *Getting research findings into practice.* BMJ Books, London

66   Hammacher, ER and van der Werken, C (1996). Acute neck sprain: 'whiplash' reappraised. *Injury* **27** (7), 463–466

1   Hammond, R and Mead, J (2003). *Identifying national priorities for physical therapy clinical guideline development.* In: Abstracts from 14th International WCPT Congress, Barcelona, Spain. 7–12 June 2003. World Confederation for Physical Therapy, 2003, London

89   Harder, S, Veilleux, M and Suissa, S (1998). The effect of socio-demographic and crash-related factors on the prognosis of whiplash. *Journal of Clinical Epidemiology* **51** (5), 377–384

64   Hartling, L, Brison, RJ, Ardern, C and Pickett, W (2001). Prognostic value of the Quebec classification of whiplash-associated disorders. *Spine* **26** (1), 36–41

158   Health Professions Council (2003). *Standards of proficiency – physiotherapists.* Health Professions Council, London

120   Heikkila, HV and Wenngren, BI (1998). Cervicocephalic kinesthetic sensibility, active range of cervical motion, and oculomotor function in patients with whiplash injury. *Archives of Physical Medicine & Rehabilitation* **79** (9), 1089–1094

37   Hendriks, O and Horgan, A (1996). Ultra-reiz current as an adjunct to standard physiotherapy treatment of the acute whiplash patient. *Physiotherapy Ireland* **17** (1), 3–7

189   Herrmann, C (1997). International experiences with the hospital anxiety and depression scale – a review of validation data and clinical results. *Journal of Psychosomatic Research* **42** (1), 17–41

169   Honey, P and Mumford, A (1986). *The manual of learning styles.* Printique, London

20   Hoving, JL, Koes, B, de Vet, HC, van der Windt, DAW, Assendelft, WJ, Van Mameren, H, Deville, WLJM, Pool, JJM, Scholten, RJPM and Bouter, LM (2002). Manual therapy, physical therapy, or continued care by a general practitioner for patients with neck pain: A randomized controlled trial. *Annals of Internal Medicine* **136**, 713–722

174   Huijbregts, MP, Myers, AM, Kay, TM and Gavin, TS (2002). Systematic outcome measurement in clinical practice: challenges experienced by physiotherapists. *Physiotherapy Canada* **54** (1), 25–31, 36

23   Humphreys, BK and Irgens, PM (2002). The effect of a rehabilitation exercise program on head repositioning accuracy and reported levels of pain in chronic neck pain subjects. *Journal of Whiplash and Related Disorders* **1**, 99–112

21   Hurwitz, EL, Morgenstern, H, Harber, P, Kominski, GF, Yu, F and Adams, AH (2002). A randomized trial of chiropractic manipulation and mobilization for patients with neck pain: Clinical outcomes from the UCLA neck-pain study. *American Journal of Public Health* **92**, 1634–1641

175   Huskisson, EC (1974). Measurement of pain. *Lancet* **2** (7889), 1127–1131

154   Irnich, D, Behrens, N, Molzen, H, Konig, A, Gleditsch, J, Krauss, M, Natalis, M, Senn, E, Beyer, A and Schops, P (2001). Randomised trial of acupuncture compared with conventional massage and "sham" laser acupuncture for treatment of chronic neck pain. *British Medical Journal* **322** (7302), 1574–1578

79   Jakobsson, L, Lundell, B, Norin, H and Isaksson Hellman, I (2000). WHIPS – Volvo's whiplash protection study. *Accident Analysis and Prevention* **32** (2), 307–319

162   Jensen, GM and Lorish, CD (1994). Promoting patient cooperation with exercise programs: linking research, theory, and practice. *Arthritis Care and Research* **7** (4), 181–189

132   Jull, G (2000). Deep cervical flexor muscle dysfunction in whiplash. World Congress on whiplash-associated disorders in Vancouver, British Columbia, Canada. February 1999. *Journal of Musculoskeletal Pain* **8** (1–2), 143–154

17   Jull, G (2001). For self-perceived benefit from treatment for chronic neck pain, multimodal treatment is more effective than home exercises, and both are more effective than advice alone. *Australian Journal of Physiotherapy* **47** (3), 215

145   Karjalainen, K, Malmivaara, A, van Tulder, M, Roine, R, Jauhiainen, M, Hurri, H and Koes, B (2003a). *Multidisciplinary biopsychosocial rehabilitation for subacute low back pain among working age adults.* The Cochrane Library: Update Software, Oxford

155   Karjalainen, K, Malmivaara, A, van Tulder, M, Roine, R, Jauhiainen, M, Hurri, H and Koes, B (2003b). *Multidisciplinary biopsychosocial rehabilitation for neck and shoulder pain among working age adults.* The Cochrane Library: Update Software, Oxford

67   Karlsborg, M, Smed, A, Jespersen, H, Stephensen, S, Cortsen, M, Jennum, P, Herning, M, Korfitsen, E and Werdelin, L (1997). A prospective study of 39 patients with whiplash injury. *Acta Neurologica Scandinavica* **95** (2), 65–72

101   Kendall, NAS, Linton, SJ and Main, CJ (1997). *Guide to assessing psychological yellow flags in acute low back pain: risk factors for long term disability and work loss.* Accident Rehabilitation & Compensation Insursance Corporation of New Zealand and the National Health Committee, Wellington

28   Kjellman, G and Oberg, B (2002). A randomized clinical trial comparing general exercise, McKenzie treatment and a control group in patients with neck pain. *Journal of Rehabilitation Medicine* **34** (4), 183–190

141   Kjellman, G, Skargren, EI and Oberg, BE (1999). A critical analysis of randomised clinical trials on neck pain and treatment efficacy. A review of the literature. *Scandinavian Journal of Rehabilitation Medicine* **31** (3), 139–152

167   Knowles, M (1983). The modern practice of adult education from pedagogy to androgogy. In: Tight, MM, ed., *Adult learning and education*, pp. 53–70. Croom Helm in association with the Open University, London

113   Koelbaek Johansen, M, Graven-Nielsen, T, Schou Olesen, A and Arendt-Nielsen, L (1999). Generalised muscular hyperalgesia in chronic whiplash syndrome. *Pain* **83** (2), 229–234

22   Korthals-de Bos, IB, Hoving, JL, van Tulder, M, Rutten-van Molken, MP, Ader, HJ, de Vet, HC, Koes, B, Vondeling, H and Bouter, LM (2003). Cost effectiveness of physiotherapy, manual therapy, and general practitioner care for neck pain: economic evaluation alongside a randomised controlled trial. *British Medical Journal* **326** (7395), 911–914

18   Kwan, O and Friel, J (2003). Management of chronic pain in whiplash injury. *Journal of Bone & Joint Surgery – British Volume* **85b** (6), 931–932

112   Lord, S, Barnsley, L, Wallis, BJ and Bogduk, N (1996). Chronic cervical zygapophysial joint pain after whiplash: a placebo-controlled prevalence study. *Spine* **21** (15), 1737–1745

133   Loudon, JK, Ruhl, M and Field, E (1997). Ability to reproduce head position after whiplash injury. *Spine* **22** (8), 865–868

126   Magee, DJ (1997). *Orthopaedic physical assessment*. Saunders, New York

15   Magee, DJ, Oborn-Barrett, E, Turner, S and Fenning, N (2000). A systematic overview of the effectiveness of physical therapy intervention on soft tissue neck injury following trauma. *Physiotherapy Canada* **52** (2), 111–130

47   Maher, CG, Sherrington, C, Herbert, RD, Moseley, AM and Elkins, M (2003). Reliability of the PEDro scale for rating quality of randomized controlled trials. *Physical Therapy* **83** (8), 713–721

104   Maimaris, C, Barnes, MR and Allen, MJ (1988). 'Whiplash injuries' of the neck: a retrospective study. *Injury* **19** (6), 393–396

108   Main, CJ and Burton, AK (2000). Economic and occupational influences on pain and disability. In: Main, CJ and Spanswick, CS, eds. *Pain management – An interdisciplinary approach*, pp. 63–87. Churchill Livingstone, London

96   Main, CJ and Watson, PJ (1999). Psychological aspects of pain. *Manual Therapy* **4** (4), 203–215

129   Maitland, GD, Hengeveld, E and Banks, K (2001). *Maitland's vertebral manipulation*. Butterworth Heinmann, Oxford

136   Matsumoto, M, Fujimura, Y, Suzuki, N, Toyama, Y and Shiga, H (1998). Cervical curvature in acute whiplash injuries: prospective comparative study with asymptomatic subjects. *Injury* **29** (10), 775–778

110   Mayou, R and Radanov, BP (1996). Whiplash neck injury. *Journal of Psychosomatic Research* **40** (5), 461–474

12   McClune, T, Burton, AK and Waddell, G (2002). Whiplash associated disorders: a review of the literature to guide patient information and advice. *Emergency Medical Journal: EMJ* **19** (6), 499–506

53   McKenna, HP (1994). The Delphi technique: a worthwhile research approach for nursing? *Journal of Advanced Nursing* **19** (6), 1221–1225

39   McKinney, LA (1989). Early mobilisation and outcome in acute sprains of the neck. *British Medical Journal* **299** (6706), 1006–1008

38   McKinney, LA, Dornan, JO and Ryan, M (1989). The role of physiotherapy in the management of acute neck sprains following road-traffic accidents. *Archives of Emergency Medicine* **6** (1), 27–33

90   McLean, AJ (1995). Neck injury severity and vehicle design. In *Biomechanics of neck injury*. Proceedings of a seminar held in Adelaide, Australia pp 47–50. NH&MRC Road Accident Research Unit, University of Adelaide. Institution of Engineers, Canberra

19   Meal, G (2002). A clinical trial investigating the possible effect of the supine cervical rotary manipulation and the supine rotary break manipulation in the treatment of mechanical neck pain: a pilot study. *Journal of Manipulative & Physiological Therapeutics* **25** (8), 541–542

40   Mealy, K, Brennan, H and Fenelon, GC (1986). Early mobilization of acute whiplash injuries. *British Medical Journal (Clinical Research edition)* **292** (6521), 656–657

4   Mills, H and Horne, G (1986). Whiplash – manmade disease? *New Zealand Medical Journal* **99** (802), 373–374

152   Mior, S (2001). Manipulation and mobilization in the treatment of chronic pain. *Clinical Journal of Pain* **17** (4) Supplement: S70–76

202   Mondloch, MV, Cole, DC and Frank, JW (2001). Does how you do depend on how you think you'll do? A systematic review of the evidence for a relation between patients' recovery expectations and health outcomes. *Canadian Medical Association Journal* **165** (2), 174–179

166   Moore, A and Jull, G (2001). The art of listening. *Manual Therapy* **6** (3)

168   Moore, A, Hilton, R, Morris, J, Calladine, L and Bristow, H (1997). *The clinical educator – role development*. Churchill Livingstone, Edinburgh

213   Motor Accidents Authority of New South Wales (2001). Guidelines for the management of whiplash associated disorders. Motor Accidents Authority of New South Wales. Available from: http://www.maa.nsw.gov.au/injury43whiplash.htm (Accessed 6th May 2005)

74   Mulhall, KJ, Moloney, M, Burke, TE and Masterson, E (2003). Chronic neck pain following road traffic accidents in an Irish setting and it's relationship to seat belt use and low back pain. *Irish Medical Journal* **96** (2), 53–54

49   Murphy, MK, Black, NA, Lamping, DL, McKee, CM, Sanderson, CFB, Ashkam, J and Marteau, T (1998). Consensus development methods and their use in clinical guideline development. *In Health Technologies Assessment* **2** (3). Available from http://www.mrw.interscience.wiley.com/cochrane/clhta/aricles/HTA-988414/frame.html (Accessed 3rd June 2005)

8   Office for National Statistics (2002). *Road accident casualties: by road user type and severity 1992-2002: annual abstract of statistics.* Office for National Statistics. Available from: http://www.statistics.gov.uk/STATBASE/ssdataset.asp?vlnk=4031 (Accessed 6th May 2005)

75   Otremski, I, Marsh, JL, McLardy-Smith, PD and Newman, RJ (1989). Soft tissue cervical spinal injuries in motor vehicle accidents. *Injury* **20** (6), 349–351

59   Panjabi, MM, Cholewicki, J, Nibu, K, Grauer, JN, Babat, LB and Dvorak, J (1998). Mechanism of whiplash injury. *Clinical Biomechanics* **13** (4–5), 239–249

62   Panjabi, MM, Pearson, AM, Ito, S, Ivancic, PC and Wang, JL (2004). Cervical spine curvature during simulated whiplash. *Clinical Biomechanics* **19** (1), 1–9

105   Parmar, HV and Raymakers, R (1993). Neck injuries from rear impact road traffic accidents: prognosis in persons seeking compensation. *Injury* **24** (2), 75–78

181   Paterson, C (1996). Measuring outcomes in primary care: a patient generated measure, MYMOP, compared with the SF-36 health survey. *British Medical Journal* **312** (7037), 1016–1020

41   Pennie, BH and Agambar, LJ (1990). Whiplash injuries. A trial of early management. *Journal of Bone & Joint Surgery – British Volume* **72** (2), 277–279

128   Petty, N and Moore, A (2001). *A neuromusculoskeletal examination and assessment: a handbook for therapists*. Churchill Livingstone, Edinburgh

173   Pietrobon, R, Coeytaux, RR, Carey, TS, Richardson, WJ and DeVellis, RF (2002). Standard scales for measurement of functional outcome for cervical pain or dysfunction: a systematic review. *Spine* **27** (5), 515–522

51   Pope, C and Mays, N (1999). *Qualitative research in health care*. 2nd Edition. BMJ books, London

139   PRODIGY (2001). *Prodigy clinical guidance – neck pain*. Department of Health. Available from: http://www.prodigy.nhs.uk/guidance.asp?gt=Neck%20pain (Accessed 6th May 2005)

42   Provinciali, L, Baroni, M, Illuminati, L and Ceravolo, MG (1996). Multimodal treatment to prevent the late whiplash syndrome. *Scandinavian Journal of Rehabilitation Medicine* **28** (2), 105–111

165   Richardson, K and Moran, S (1995). Developing standards for patient information. *International Journal of Health Care Quality Assurance* **8** (7), 27–31

170   Rodwell, CM (1996). An analysis of the concept of empowerment. *Journal of Advanced Nursing* **23** (2), 305–313

171   Rollnick, S, Mason, P and Butler, C (1999). *Health behaviour changes, A guide for practitioners.* Churchill Livingstone, Edinburgh

43   Rosenfeld, M, Gunnarsson, R and Borenstein, P (2000). Early intervention in whiplash-associated disorders: a comparison of two treatment protocols. *Spine* **25** (14), 1782–1787

29   Rosenfeld, M, Seferiadis, A, Carlsson, J and Gunnarsson, R (2003). Active intervention in patients with whiplash-associated disorders improves long-term prognosis: a randomized controlled clinical trial. *Spine* **28** (22), 2491–2498

205   Rousseau, N, McColl, E, Newton, J, Grimshaw, J and Eccles, M (2003). Practice based, longitudinal, qualitative interview study of computerised evidence based guidelines in primary care. *British Medical Journal* **326** (7384), 314

124   Royal College of General Practitioners (1999). *Clinical guidelines for the management of acute low back pain*. Royal College of General Practitioners, London

135   RCR Working Party (2003). *Making the best use of a department of clinical radiology, guidelines for doctors, 5th edition*. The Royal College of Radiologists, London

92   Ryan, GA (2000). Etiology and outcomes of whiplash: review and update. World Congress on whiplash-associated disorders, Vancouver, British Columbia, Canada. February 1999. *Journal of Musculoskeletal Pain* **8** (1–2), 3–14

52   Sackman, H (1975). *Delphi critique*. Lexington Books, Lexington MA

81   Salmi, LR, Thomas, H, Fabry, JJ and Girard, R (1989). The effect of the 1979 French seatbelt law on the nature and severity of injuries to front seat occupants. *Accident Analysis and Prevention* **21**, 589–594

144   Sarig-Bahat, H (2003). Evidence for exercise therapy in mechanical neck disorders. *Manual Therapy* **8** (1), 10–20

121   Schmand, B, Lindeboom, J, Schagen, S, Heijt, R, Koene, T and Hamburger, HL (1998). Cognitive complaints in patients after whiplash injury: the impact of malingering. *Journal of Neurology, Neurosurgery, and Psychiatry* **64** (3), 339–343

103   Schofferman, J and Wasserman, S (1994). Successful treatment of low back pain and neck pain after a motor vehicle accident despite litigation. *Spine* **19** (9), 1007–1010

77   Scholten-Peeters, GG, Verhagen, AP, Bekkering, GE, van der Windt, DA, Barnsley, L, Oostendorp, RA and Hendriks, EJ (2003). Prognostic factors of whiplash-associated disorders: a systematic review of prospective cohort studies. *Pain* **104** (1–2), 303–322

6   Scholten-Peeters, GGM, Bekkering, GE, Verhagen, AP, van der Windt, DAW, Lanser, K, Hendriks, EJM and Oostendorp, RA (2002). Clinical practice guideline for the physiotherapy of patients with whiplash-associated disorders. *Spine* **27** (4), 412–422

26   Scholten-Peeters, GGM, Verhagen, AP, Neeleman-van der Steen, CW, Hurkmans, JC, Wams, RW and Oostendorp, RA (2003). Randomized clinical trial of conservative treatment for patients with whiplash-associated disorders: considerations for the design and dynamic treatment protocol. *Journal of Manipulative & Physiological Therapeutics* **26** (7), 412–420

117   Schrader, H, Obelieniene, D and Ferrari, R (2000). Temporomandibular and whiplash injury in Lithuania. World Congress on whiplash-associated disorders, Vancouver, British Columbia, Canada. February 1999. *Journal of Musculoskeletal Pain* **8** (1–2), 133–142

88   Schrader, H, Obelieniene, D, Bovim, G, Surkiene, D, Mickeviciene, D, Miseviciene, I and Sand, T (1996). Natural evolution of late whiplash syndrome outside the medicolegal context. *Lancet* **347** (9010), 1207–1211

76   Schuller, E, Eisenmenger, W and Beier, G (2000). Whiplash injury in low speed car accidents: assessment of biomechanical cervical spine loading and injury prevention in a forensic sample. World Congress on whiplash-associated disorders, Vancouver, British Columbia, Canada. February 1999. *Journal of Musculoskeletal Pain* **8** (1–2), 55–67

11   Scottish Intercollegiate Guidelines Network (2001). *Sign 50: A guideline developers' handbook.* Scottish Intercollegiate Guidelines Network. Available from: http://www.sign.ac.uk/guidelines/fulltext/50/index.html (Accessed 3rd June 2005)

153   Smith, LA, Oldman, AD, McQuay, HJ and Moore, RA (2000). Teasing apart quality and validity in systematic reviews: an example from acupuncture trials in chronic neck and back pain. *Pain* **86** (1-2), 119–132

70   Soderlund, A and Lindberg, P (1999). Long-term functional and psychological problems in whiplash associated disorders. *International Journal of Rehabilitation Research* **22** (2), 77–84

44   Soderlund, A, Olerud, C and Lindberg, P (2000). Acute whiplash-associated disorders (WAD): the effects of early mobilization and prognostic factors in long-term symptomatology. *Clinical Rehabilitation* **14** (5), 457–467

2   Spitzer, WO, Skovron, ML, Salmi, LR, Cassidy, JD, Duranceau, J, Suissa, S, Zeiss, E, Weinstein, JN and Nogbuk, N (1995). Scientific monograph of the Quebec Task Force on whiplash-associated disorders: Redefining 'Whiplash' and its management. *Spine* **20** (8)

72   Squires, B, Gargan, MF and Bannister, GC (1996). Soft-tissue injuries of the cervical spine. 15-year follow-up. *Journal of Bone & Joint Surgery – British Volume* **78** (6), 955–957

107   Sterling, M, Kenardy, J, Jull, G and Vicenzino, B (2003). The development of psychological changes following whiplash injury. *Pain* **106** (3), 481–489

86   Sterner, Y, Toolanen, G, Gerdle, B and Hildingsson, C (2003). The incidence of whiplash trauma and the effects of different factors on recovery. *Journal of Spinal Disorders & Techniques* **16** (2), 195–199

143   Stevinson, C and Ernst, E (2002). Risks associated with spinal manipulation. *American Journal of Medicine* **112** (7), 566–571

160   Stewart, M and Roter, D (1989). *Communicating with medical patients.* Sage Publications, New York.

178   Stratford, PW, Riddle, DL, Binkley, JM, Spadoni, G, Westaway, MD and Padfield, B (1999). Using the Neck Disability Index to make decisions concerning individual patients. *Physiotherapy Canada* **51** (2), 107–112

73   Suissa, S, Harder, S and Veilleux, M (2001). The relation between initial symptoms and signs and the prognosis of whiplash. *European Spine Journal* **10** (1), 44–49

71   Sullivan, MJ, Hall, E, Bartolacci, R, Sullivan, ME and Adams, H (2002). Perceived cognitive deficits, emotional distress and disability following whiplash injury. *Pain Research & Management* **7** (3), 120–126

184   Swinkels-Meewisse, EJ, Swinkels, RA, Verbeek, AL, Vlaeyen, JW and Oostendorp, RA (2003). Psychometric properties of the Tampa Scale for kinesiophobia and the fear-avoidance beliefs questionnaire in acute low back pain. *Manual Therapy* **8** (1), 29–36

98   Symonds, TL, Burton, AK, Tillotson, KM and Main, CJ (1996). Do attitudes and beliefs influence work loss due to low back trouble? *Occupational Medicine* **46** (1), 25–32

63   Tenenbaum, A, Rivano Fischer, M, Tjell, C, Edblom, M and Sunnerhagen, KS (2002). The Quebec classification and a new Swedish classification for whiplash-associated disorders in relation to life satisfaction in patients at high risk of chronic functional impairment and disability. *Journal of Rehabilitation Medicine* **34** (3), 114–118

203   Thomas, E, Croft, PR, Paterson, SM, Dziedzic, K and Hay, EM (2004). What influences participants' treatment preference and can it influence outcome? Results from a primary care-based randomised trial for shoulder pain. *British Journal of General Practice* **54** (499), 93–96

30   Thuile, C and Walzl, M (2002). Evaluation of electromagnetic fields in the treatment of pain in patients with lumbar radiculopathy or the whiplash syndrome. *Neurorehabilitation* **17**, 63–67

83   Tunbridge, RJ (1990). The long term effect of seat belt legislation on road user injury patterns. *Health Bulletin (Edinburgh)* **48** (6), 347–349

192   Upadhyaya, AK and Stanley, I (1993). Hospital anxiety depression scale. *British Journal of General Practice* **43** (373), 349–350

148   van der Heijden, GJ, Beurskens, AJ, Koes, B, Assendelft, WJ, de Vet, HC and Bouter, LM (1995). The efficacy of traction for back and neck pain: a systematic, blinded review of randomized clinical trial methods. *Physical Therapy* **75** (2), 93–104

204   van Tulder, M, Kovacs, F, Muller, G, Airaksinen, O, Balague, F, Broos, L, Burton, K, Gil del Real, MT, Hanninen, O, Henrotin, Y, Hildebrandt, J, Indahl, A, Leclerc, A, Manniche, C, Tilscher, H, Ursin, H, Vleeming, A and Zanoli, G (2002). European guidelines for the management of low back pain. *Acta Orthopaedica Scandinavica* **73** (305), 20–25

24   Vendrig, AA, van Akkerveeken, PF and McWhorter, KR (2000). Results of a multimodal treatment program for patients with chronic symptoms after a whiplash injury of the neck. *Spine* **25** (2), 238–244

46   Verhagen, AP, de Vet, HC, de Bie, RA, Kessels, AG, Boers, M, Bouter, LM and Knipschild, PG (1998). The Delphi list: a criteria list for quality assessment of randomized clinical trials for conducting systematic reviews developed by Delphi consensus. *Journal of Clinical Epidemiology* **51** (12), 1235–1241

13   Verhagen, AP, Peeters, GGM, de Bie, RA and Oostendorp, RA (2002). Conservative treatment for whiplash. *The Cochrane Library: Update Software, Oxford*

177   Vernon, H (1996). The Neck Disability Index: patient assessment and outcome monitoring in whiplash. *Journal of Musculoskeletal Pain* **4** (4), 95–104

179   Vernon, H (2000). Assessment of self-rated disability, impairment, and sincerity of effort in whiplash-associated disorder. *Journal of Musculoskeletal Pain* **8**, 1–2

176   Vernon, H and Mior, S (1991). The Neck Disability Index: a study of reliability and validity. *Journal of Manipulative Physiological Therapeutics* **14** (7), 409–415

91   Versteegen, GJ, Kingma, J, Meijler, WJ and ten Duis, HJ (1998). Neck sprain in patients injured in car accidents: a retrospective study covering the period 1970–1994. *European Spine Journal* **7** (3), 195–200

85   Versteegen, GJ, Kingma, J, Meijler, WJ and ten Duis, HJ (2000). Neck sprain after motor vehicle accidents in drivers and passengers. *European Spine Journal* **9** (6), 547–552

182   Vlaeyen, J, Kole-Snijders, A, Boeren, R, van Eek, H (1995). Fear of movement/(re)injury in chronic low back pain and its relation to behavioural performance. *Pain* **62**, 363–372

102   Waddell, G (1998). *The back pain revolution.* Churchill Livingstone, Edinburgh

99   Waddell, G and Burton, AK (2001). Occupational health guidelines for the management of low back pain at work: evidence review. *Occupational Medicine* **51** (2), 124–135

95   Waddell, G and Main, CJ (1984). Assessment of severity in low-back disorders. *Spine* **9** (2), 204–208

78   Waddell, G, Burton, AK and McClune, T (2001). *The whiplash book.* The Stationery Office, Norwich.

60   Walz, FH and Muser, MH (2000). Biomechanical assessment of soft tissue cervical spine disorders and expert opinion in low speed collisions. *Accident Analysis and Prevention* **32** (2), 161–165

25   Wang, WT, Olson, SL, Campbell, AH, Hanten, WP and Gleeson, PB (2003). Effectiveness of physical therapy for patients with neck pain: an individualized approach using a clinical decision-making algorithm. *American Journal of Physical Medicine & Rehabilitation* **82** (3), 203–218

97   Watson, PJ (1999). Psychosocial assessment: the emergence of a new fashion, or a new tool in physiotherapy for musculoskeletal pain? *Physiotherapy* **85** (10), 533–535

210   Wensing, M, van der Weijden, T and Grol, R (1998). Implementing guidelines and innovations in general practice: which interventions are effective? *British Journal of General Practice* **48** (427), 991–997

180   Westaway, MD, Stratford, PW and Binkley, JM (1998). The patient-specific functional scale: validation of its use in persons with neck dysfunction. *Journal of Orthopaedic and Sports Physical Therapy* **27** (5), 331–338

146   White, AR and Ernst, E (1999). A systematic review of randomized controlled trials of acupuncture for neck pain. *Rheumatology* **38** (2), 143–147

185   Woby, SR, Roach, NK, Watson, PJ, Birch, KM and Urmston, M (2002). A further analysis of the psychometric properties of the Tampa Scale for Kinesiophobia (TSK). *Journal of Bone & Joint Surgery – British Volume* **84-B (Supp III)** (49)

186   Woby, SR, Watson, PJ, Roach, NK and Urmston, M (2003). *Psychometric properties of the Tampa scale for kinesiophobia.* Poster in 4th Congress of The European Federation of the International Association for the Study of Pain Chapters (Pain in Europe IV), Prague, Czech Rebublic. September 2003

31   Wood, TG, Colloca, CJ and Matthews, R (2001). A pilot randomized clinical trial on the relative effect of instrumental (MFMA) versus manual (HVLA) manipulation in the treatment of cervical spine dysfunction. *Journal of Manipulative & Physiological Therapeutics* **24** (4), 260–271

131   Yeung, E, Jones, M and Hall, B (1997). The response to the slump test in a group of female whiplash patients. *Australian Journal of Physiotherapy* **43** (4), 245–252

188   Zigmond, AS and Snaith, RP (1983). The hospital anxiety and depression scale. *Acta Psychiatrica Scandinavica* **67** (6), 361–370